DEALING WITH DEMENTIA

Recent European Research

DAVID F. MARKS is Professor of Psychology and the Head of Health Research Centre at Middlesex University. David Marks has taught or conducted research in England, Italy, New Zealand, Norway, Spain and the USA and authored more than 250 research publications, including 11 books. He was a partner and project leader in the European Alzheimer's Clearing House (E.A.C.H.) for two years.

CATHERINE M. SYKES is a Research Officer and Chartered Health Psychologist who has co-ordinated research projects at the Health Research Centre, Middlesex University for 4 years. Catherine Sykes has worked on several Alzheimer's Disease projects including a study of the determinants of carer burden and an investigation of good practice of Alzheimer's services in the European Union.

Other titles in the Middlesex University's Health Series include:

Caersarean Birth in Britain
Improving the Health of the Nation
Improving Men's Health

Series Editor: Colin Francome

DEALING WITH DEMENTIA
Recent European Research

DAVID F. MARKS AND CATHERINE M. SYKES

Middlesex University Press
London, England

First published in 2000 by Middlesex University Press

Middlesex University Press is an imprint of Middlesex University
Services Limited, Bounds Green Road, London N11 2NQ

A CIP catalogue record for this book is available from The British Library

ISBN 1 898253 32 3

Financed with the assistance of the European Community
(SOC 97 201318 05F03)

Designed by Elizabeth Durrant from a diskette supplied by the authors.
Manufacture coordinated in UK by Book in Hand Limited, London N6 5AH.

Contents

PREFACE AND ACKNOWLEDGEMENTS

This book is a synthesis of recent European research on dementia care. It is directed towards informal carers, health professionals, journalists and policy makers. The book has three objectives: (1) To discuss in the plainest possible language one of the most significant social questions of the contemporary world - how are we going to deal with the increasing problem of dementia? (2) To bring together in one place the information, conclusions and recommendations from thirty-four projects supported by the European Commission. (3) To help raise public awareness about facts concerning dementia, especially the facts that dementia is the end product of disease, not an inevitable feature of ageing, and that the problem is increasing dramatically.

Part One introduces the field of dementia. The main medical conditions associated with dementia symptoms and changes are described. We then briefly discuss theories of the causes of Alzheimer's disease, one of the main conditions associated with dementia. The methods used in assessment and diagnosis are described. Recent data on prevalence and incidence, and known risk factors are summarised. Part Two summarises and discusses recent European research on dementia care drawn principally from 34 projects co-funded by the European Commission Directorate-General V (EC DG V) in 1995 and 1996. We discuss the new findings from these projects under these headings: informal care, formal care, communication and information, treatments and interventions, policy and equity, and the future. Part Three presents a brief outline of the 34 projects, some final conclusions concerning the methodology and management of projects of this kind, Alzheimer Europe's declaration of the needs and rights of people with dementia and their carers and a recommendation to the European Commission. The book ends with a glossary of terms, bibliography, and addresses of relevant organisations.

We do not attempt to cover all aspects of dementia, only those topics that were the focus of the EC DG V Alzheimer's projects in 1995-6, together with other necessary information concerning the nature of dementia and its treatment. We have been unable to include much of the recent research on the causes of Alzheimer's disease and other forms of dementia. We have tried to write in as reader-friendly a style as possible. In places, however, it has been impossible to avoid scientific or health care terminology. The Glossary enables the reader to check the definition and meaning of all key words.

Each project is referred to in the text by number as listed in the project summaries in Chapter 11. Project numbers are shown in superscript as [1], [2], [3] etc. All project leaders were sent a copy of the manuscript before publication so that they could check the accuracy of the information presented. Nearly 50 individuals, all expert on some aspect of dementia, were able to read and comment on this book before it went to press. We are therefore hopeful that it represents in a factually accurate way the current information on this topic as this particularly relates to the situation in Europe. Final responsibility for the information and its synthesis in this particular form of course rests with us, the authors.

The research for this book was conducted with the financial support of the European Community (SOC97 201318 05F03).

We thank Lars Rasmussen of DG V, Luxembourg, for his personal help and support at all stages of this project. We acknowledge the support of the European Alzheimer Clearing House (EACH) in Brussels. In particular we thank Professor Franz Baro and Mrs Leen Meulenbergs. Helpful discussion and advice were provided at different times and places by Professor Mary Marshall of the Dementia Services Development Centre at the University of Stirling, Scotland, Professor Hervé Allain at the Université de Rennes, France, and Jean George of Alzheimer Europe, Luxembourg.

We also thank the many EC Alzheimer's project leaders, whose project reports are cited in the text, for their co-operation and, in some cases, for allowing us to visit. This book is a synthesis of information from all of these projects seen collectively as a European-wide exercise. We hope that this book will facilitate and improve dissemination of information on dementia especially among carers, professionals, journalists, the media and policy makers.

In regard to the Middlesex/EACH study[11], we acknowledge the Alzheimer's Disease Society and its branches in London for their help in the recruitment of informal carers into our survey. We especially thank Cheryl Pitt and Sally Thomas who conducted many interviews with informal carers in a sensitive and caring manner.

We are also pleased to acknowledge the artistry of photographer Carl Cordonnier as evidenced by his wonderful photographic study of a woman with Alzheimer's reproduced on the cover. Thanks also to Elizabeth Durrant for her thoughtful illustrations and assistance in the production of the manuscript in photo-ready form for printing.

Preface and Acknowledgements

Of special importance were the many thousands of people who willingly participated in one way or another in the projects summarised here. Is it to them, and to all people with dementia and their carers, that we dedicate this book.

David F. Marks and Catherine M. Sykes

Middlesex University Health Research Centre

London, UK

July 1999

FOREWORD

In the years to come the health care systems in Europe will be put under increasing pressure and the cries for reforms will become louder. This challenges the principle of equity. The main reasons for the strains on the health care system are: (i) the population is ageing and there has been a drop in the fertility rate that means a decrease in the active population; (ii) technology is improving; and (iii) expectations are increasing. Tax increases to support this strain could be counterproductive by having a negative impact on employment and subsequently on tax revenues.

Ageing of the population is one of the most remarkable advances of modern times. In the course of this century developed countries have witnessed a dramatic increase in life expectancy. At the turn of the century it was 40-50 years; at the new millennium it has reached 75-80 years.

The second report (1996) on the demographic situation in the European Union published by the European Commission focuses on the dominant factor in our demographic future: the extent and acceleration of the ageing process. According to this report, by 2025 the number of people aged over 60 will increase by 37 million - a growth of nearly 50% to 113.5 million pensioners in the European Union, nearly one third of the population. At present, the global population aged 65 and over is increasing at a rate of more than 800,000 people per month. But the most rapid increase is taking place in the 80 years and older age group.

An imbalance in the age distribution of a population is not a new factor. What is new about the present situation is that the modified age structure of Europe's populations, as of the rest of the world, will eventually threaten the very existence of the so-called modern societies as we know them and oblige us to change. It is evident from the debate on savings in the health sector that unless we begin to change our attitudes towards ageing, we shall very soon reach the point where we see the ageing population as a "burden" and forget that older people are an asset.

The ageing population will mean a rapid increase in Alzheimer's Disease and Related Disorders (ADRD) and an increased stress on their carers. What may eventually rock the health care system are the new drugs rapidly coming into the market which can slow down the progress of Alzheimer's disease. Will society and politicians be willing to pay for a costly symptomatic treatment which will eventually lead to health costs because of higher life expectancy of these people and increased demands on institutional care?

We are told that economy rules the world and that no one can escape the laws of the maker. Anyone challenging that fanatical religion of our times is branded as irrational. Albert Jacquard in his book "L'Economie Triomphante", maintains that by following such 'economism' our humanity is running straight into the wall. 'Economism' leads inevitably to barbarism.

It is obvious that we have to determine the level of care that we are willing to provide to the older members of our population. Can society afford to go on investing in unproductive people with permanent disabilities without any hope for a cure? Should interventions be rationed or age-determined? Should they be reserved only for the fittest or the rich? Should we do the utmost to preserve human life and dignity at any cost because the human being is the essence of life? These are questions essential to the future of Western civilisation and which merit an in-depth public debate.

When the European Commission started its Alzheimer's projects in 1995, it was my firm conviction that we can and should. I believe there is a place for everyone in our society. And this philosophy has enlightened and guided the Commission's work.

We should not think in terms of economics alone. We should think of people as human beings. It is after all a question of resource allocation how wealth and production of society is to be consumed. The decrease in the active population can be made up for by increased productivity. The annual growth needed to support the dependent population is not unrealistic or unachievable. We should introduce new concepts adapted to the demands and spirit of our time.

There is a desperate need for inter and intragenerational solidarity, in our society. The modern Welfare State has turned man into an egocentric animal. The State is taking care of everyone and individuals are taking care of themselves in order to survive materially and spiritually.

In today's society there is little or no solidarity between individuals or between generations. We have apparently forgotten the Ten Commandments that say, "Love thy neighbour as thyself" and "Honour thy father and thy mother".

We all need something to believe in. Should we revive the social message of Christianity and apply it to the engineering of the society of future generations for the benefit of everyone?

The European Parliament has been concerned with deaths and

Foreword

diseases arising from the ageing population of the EU. It has called for the European Commission to submit a specific programme of measures on Alzheimer's Disease. Between the years 1994 and 1998 the European Parliament amended its budget, allocating 10 million ECUs (the European currency that predated the Euro) specifically for Alzheimer's Disease and Related Disorders. The Commission has published an annual announcement in the Official Journal of European Communities calling for proposals into work on ADRD. To date, the Commission has contributed towards the financing of at least 67 projects.

The Commission has supported this book. The book aims to review, combine and integrate all 34 projects co-financed by the Commission in the first two years, 1995-6. This book has been written in a user-friendly way in order to attract a variety of readers such as carers, policy makers, journalists, politicians and the general public. This book demonstrates the work on ADRD that the Commission is supporting and it is hoped that more people will be educated about ADRD as a result of it.

Some of the projects co-funded by the European Commission are excellent examples of the work being carried out in this field that go along way to ensuring that the individual is not forgotten. I hope that after reading this book you will realise the importance of work in the ADRD field and the importance of treating people with ADRD as people who have their own individual personalities.

Lars Rasmussen
Principal Administrator
European Commission DG V
Luxembourg
July 1999

Part One:

What is Dementia?

CHAPTER 1: ALZHEIMER'S DISEASE AND RELATED DISORDERS

Dementia

The World Health Organisation International Classification of Diseases states:

> *Dementia is a syndrome due to disease of the brain, usually of a chronic or progressive nature, in which there is a disturbance of multiple higher cortical functions, including memory, thinking, orientation, comprehension, calculation, learning capacity, language and judgement. Consciousness is not clouded. Impairments of cognitive function are commonly accompanied, and occasionally preceded by deterioration in emotional control, social behaviour or motivation.*

The most common type of dementia is *Alzheimer's disease* (AD) caused by damage and loss of brain cells. It is a natural process to lose brain cells but when a person has Alzheimer's disease the cells are lost at a much faster rate. This has a variety of confusing and disturbing effects on a person's mind and emotions that get worse over time and do not improve. AD is sometimes referred to as "a silent disease" because it begins slowly, without any outward signs, and can develop quietly for several years before anyone notices. Dementia is more common in older people but it can occur at any age. It is also more common in women than men.

Although there are many theories, the precise causes of AD are unknown. Currently, a few drugs are available that can slow down the progression of AD, but there are no effective methods of prevention and no cure. It is therefore vitally important that we learn as much as possible about the patients' experience of the illness. As a society we also need to develop our knowledge, skills, and awareness to improve the quality of life of people with dementia.

Often it is not realised that Alzheimer's Disease and Related Disorders (ADRD) can occur in both younger and older people. Early-onset Alzheimer's disease affects people between the ages of 40 and 65. Fortunately, it occurs only very rarely at younger ages than this. However other forms of dementia can affect people at this age or even younger. Early onset dementia represents almost 10% of all cases of dementia. According to North American doctors, there are more young people suffering from Alzheimer's disease these days. There is a huge difference between the situation of older patients over 65 and younger patients. Whereas older people with dementia approach or have passed retirement age, younger people with dementia face other kinds of problems, such as giving up their jobs and family responsibilities. They also have different care needs.

A report on early onset dementia from the European Alzheimer's Clearing House (EACH)[11] conducted by Alzheimer Europe noted that only a few national Alzheimer's associations have designed services for younger sufferers. There is an almost total lack of adequate services for this group of people. This is probably due to a lack of awareness and the perception that it is not really important.

People with dementia have problems with their memory, especially their short-term memory. They forget things they have just done or said, yet they may vividly remember events from years ago. They lose their sense of time and place and become confused. New information and new things are difficult for people with dementia. As dementia gradually progresses, everyday tasks such as washing, eating and dressing slowly become impossible to perform without help. Behavioural and communication problems are also likely to arise and the person loses his or her sense of identity. Eventually twenty-four hour care is needed for the person with dementia.

Dementia must be distinguished from delirium that is an acute state of confusion. Delirium may be manifested in older people who have infections, high fever, drug reactions, bad diets, shock or constipation. These conditions demand immediate medical assessment and treatment. Mary Marshall (1990) points out that it is "crucially important to differentiate between confusion and dementia, because confusion may be a symptom of both delirium and dementia." Delirium happens suddenly whereas dementia generally develops gradually.

According to recent figures from the Erasmus University Medical School in the Netherlands[14], AD accounts for seventy percent of all cases of dementia in Europe. Because Alzheimer's disease is the most common form of dementia, most research has concentrated on this. However other related forms of dementia must also be considered. The next most common type of dementia is Multi-Infarct Dementia (MID). This is caused by a series of minor strokes that gradually affect the functioning of the brain.

Sometimes the term "Alzheimer's disease" is erroneously used to cover all forms of dementia. In fact there is a huge number of different conditions falling within dementia (or ADRD) and these are only distinguished and diagnosed with some difficulty. Before describing Alzheimer's disease in more detail, we will briefly describe the other major forms of dementia.

Multi-Infarct Dementia

In spite of the different causes, multi-infarct dementia and Alzheimer's disease can be almost impossible to tell apart clinically and are often mis-diagnosed. Multi-infarct dementia (MID) is caused by several mini strokes or infarcts. It is also referred to as "vascular dementia". When a person has a stroke, there is a blockage of an artery supplying blood to part of the brain. The lack of blood may cause nerve cells to die.

This cell death produces different deficits depending on which region of the brain has been affected. The mini strokes that cause vascular dementia often do not cause immediate deficits although they may cause some temporary confusion. It is the cumulative effect of mini strokes that usually causes vascular dementia. The strokes themselves often occur because of high blood pressure or blood clots. The symptoms of vascular dementia are similar to other forms of dementia by indicating a loss of short-term memory and a progressive decline in other abilities. In vascular dementia, however, the memory loss is more variable than in Alzheimer's disease. It often seems that the memory is not worsening as memory loss occurs with each new stroke in a series of steps.

People with vascular dementia also seem to be more aware of their condition than people with Alzheimer's disease and can learn a few strategies for dealing with it. For example, one person who knew lots of people who regularly visited the family home would habitually say, "How are **you** today?" whether or not he really could remember who they were! Despite the fact that personality seems to be relatively conserved in vascular dementia there is an increased unpredictability of the patient's behaviour.

Other forms of dementia include:

a) Creutzfeldt-Jakob disease (CJD)

Creutzfeldt-Jakob Disease (CJD) is a rare type of dementia resulting from infectious agents. It can occur at any age. Although some of the early signs of CJD are similar to Alzheimer's disease, CJD progresses much more rapidly. A person with CJD usually dies within a year. A new variant of CJD that has received considerable publicity in recent years is caused by the ingestion of meat products contaminated by *bovine spongiform encephalopathy* (BSE) popularly known as "Mad Cow disease". The disease is preventable by the avoidance of cross-contamination in the food chain.

b) Pick's disease

Pick's disease is also a rare type of dementia. It usually develops when a person is in their forties or fifties. It has a genetic cause and runs in families. It is mainly the frontal lobes of the brain that are affected in Pick's disease (see Figure 1.1). This causes a person to become apathetic and withdrawn and also their personality may change. Another main feature of Pick's disease is difficulty with expression. This is due to the fact that the area of the brain called Broca's area, which is involved in speech, is often affected. A progressive decline occurs leading to death between five and ten years after diagnosis.

c) Huntington's disease (HD)

This is another rare form of dementia, originally known as Huntington's chorea, which is inherited. A person with *Huntington's disease* not only has problems with mental deterioration but also in controlling their body movements. Their movement problems are characterised as "dancelike" and consist of uncontrollable twitching and spasms of the muscles. This disease is hereditary. Signs of Huntington's disease usually start when people are in their thirties, forties or fifties. The early signs may be either mental or physical symptoms. There is a gradual loss of memory and concentration that leads to severe dementia. HD is caused by regional loss of neurones and brain shrinkage. People at risk can have genetic counselling and then, if they wish, genetic testing to determine whether they have inherited the gene responsible for the disease.

d) AIDS-related dementia

Dementia can occur in people with AIDS due to a direct effect of the HIV virus on the brain or to infections or tumours in the brain that develop because of a low immunity.

e) Lewy-body disease

Lewy-body disease is similar to Alzheimer's disease. However unlike Alzheimer's disease this condition will vary from day to day. Short episodes of confusion may occur but will then settle. This may make care more difficult as behaviour is unpredictable. People with Lewy-body disease need to avoid drugs known as antipsychotic or neuroleptic drugs. Examples include chlorpromazine (Largactil) and thioridazine (Malarial).

f) Parkinson's disease (PD)

About 25 percent of PD patients suffer mental decline that is sufficiently severe to prevent them from remaining independent. Changes in the brain resemble those of AD and include plaques and tangles in the cortex and reduction of choline acetyltransferase (ChAT).

g) Alcoholic dementia

Alcohol damages the nervous system by causing vitamin deficiencies. The Wrench-Korsakoff's syndrome results from thiamine deficiency and causes ocular disturbances, ataxia and confusion. If it develops into a chronic disease it leads to Korsakoff's psychosis which involves a loss of short-term memory (anterograde

Figure 1.1:   Location of the lobes of the brain

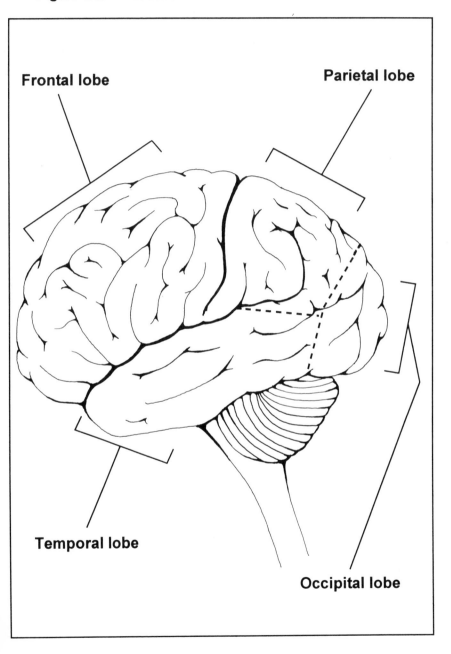

Frontal lobe

Parietal lobe

Temporal lobe

Occipital lobe

amnesia) and is irreversible. However it can be prevented by ensuring adequate thiamine intake is maintained in alcoholics.

Senile dementia

In the past, the term *senile dementia* was used to describe what was in fact Alzheimer's disease. This term was used when people lost their memory in old age. A distinction was made based on age. Senile dementia was used to describe the condition in older people (65+) while younger people were described as having "pre-senile dementia". Autopsies on the brain of people with senile dementia, carried out in the 1960s and 1970s showed characteristic features of Alzheimer's disease. It then became usual to refer to these people as *suffering from senile dementia of the Alzheimer type* (SDAT). Today these terms are discouraged, as they can be misleading. The term "a person with Alzheimer's Disease" is encouraged and generally regarded the most appropriate term by people dealing with people with Alzheimer's disease.

Yet confusion of terminology still exists, especially when translated into different languages. The Training, Teaching and Support Group (TTS Group)[5] explain in their training programme why this is important:

> *Talking about the demented person implies the mix of the illness "dementia" and the "person" who has dementia. It seems that in the statement "the demented person" the person is more or less defined by and reduced to his illness. Whereas in the statement "person having dementia" his illness is one aspect of his life and being, but the person still exists as a self-identified subject.*

Alzheimer's disease

Alzheimer's disease obtained its name from a German neurologist, Dr Alois Alzheimer (1864-1915). In 1907 Alzheimer observed changes in the brain tissue of a fifty-one year old woman who died of an unusual mental illness. This woman started showing jealously toward her husband and soon experienced memory loss. She could not find her way around her own apartment. She carried objects back and forth and would hide them. Sometimes she would cry out very loudly. It is now known that the changes in the brain tissue of this woman are the characteristic features of Alzheimer's disease and causes the symptoms of this dementia.

Alzheimer's disease is a progressive neurodegenerative disorder. This means that the cells in the brain of a person with Alzheimer's disease are slowly and progressively destroyed. Post-mortem examination of the brain in patients with AD show atrophy or shrinkage of the brain resulting from considerable cell loss. Microscopic examination of brain tissue reveals extensive occurrence of plaques and tangles (see next Chapter for more details). It is not a contagious disease.

The early stages of AD are associated with minimal changes in thinking and memory that are noticeable as "mild cognitive impairment" (MCI). Considerable efforts are being made to improve our ability make early detection and diagnosis.

The common symptoms of Alzheimer's disease fall into five categories:

1) Memory

Many of the problems that a person with Alzheimer's disease encounters are related to memory loss in some way. For example forgetting to eat, forgetting where the toilet is or forgetting who their carer is. Memory loss is often one of the first signs that lead family or friends to suspect Alzheimer's disease.

Forgetting things just said or done is a major symptom of Alzheimer's disease. This is often referred to as problems with short-term memory. Events that happened in the past often remain clear for people in the early stages of Alzheimer's disease. So, for example, someone may not remember that they have just had a cup of tea but they may remember a present that they received for their tenth birthday.

With memory problems comes a loss of sense of time. People with Alzheimer's disease often have difficulty judging what time of day it is. The passing of time also is a problem. It may be difficult for them to judge whether five minutes has passed or five hours.

People with Alzheimer's disease have difficulty telling the time quite early on in the disease. When asked the time they might be able to read the clock correctly but they may not understand the significance of time. In some cases the significance of time is understood but the answer, when time is given, is forgotten and the question 'What time is it?" is constantly repeated.

Not having a sense of time can cause a lot of worry for the person with Alzheimer's disease. They may worry that they have been deserted or that they are late. This lack of sense of time is often accompanied by disturbances in the internal clock. For example they may no longer feel naturally tired in the evening and sleeping patterns may become disturbed.

2) Verbal and Non-Verbal Communication

When a person has Alzheimer's disease their ability to speak, to be understood and to understand others gradually deteriorate. Difficulty or loss of the ability to understand spoken or written language is sometimes referred to as "aphasia"

Problems with verbal communication can cause frustration, confusion or anger. A person with Alzheimer's disease may have needs and wishes that are not met due to communication problems. Others may misunderstand their behaviour and this may lead to feelings of isolation.

During conversations, a person with Alzheimer's disease may fail to look at a person when they are talking to them. She may interrupt when another person is talking or alternatively may remain silent when a comment or response is expected. Non-verbal clues such as eye contact and shifting of posture become difficult to interpret when someone has Alzheimer's disease.

3) Changes in Mood

People with Alzheimer's disease quite often have abrupt changes of mood. One moment they may be happy and the next moment they are sad. At times, these changes can be quite dramatic. Such sudden changes of mood are due to the illness rather than a reaction against something.

People with Alzheimer's may also experience apathy or indifference. They may, for example, sit in a chair for hours, not doing anything, not reacting and not speaking. They seem to not care about anything. This can be very distressing for carers. They may think the person they are caring for is being deliberately difficult. However, this is a common manifestation of the disease.

People with Alzheimer's disease may experience depression to the point that it becomes a medical problem. It may be difficult to tell the difference between depression and the symptoms of Alzheimer's disease as many of the symptoms are the same, e.g. loss of motivation, decreased energy and sleep disturbances. The main symptoms of depression include a depressed mood, loss of interest or pleasure, altered appetite, sleep disturbance, fatigue, agitation, feelings of guilt and worthlessness and suicidal thoughts. Not all of these symptoms have to be present for a person to be classed as having depression. These symptoms are sometimes accompanied by other symptoms such as tearfulness, anxiety and headaches and pains. Depression is not a necessary part of dementia and depressive symptoms in people with dementia are treatable.

4) Problems with Daily Life
Assistance with everyday tasks such as tasks related to personal hygiene is needed when a person has Alzheimer's disease. As Alzheimer's disease progresses the person may lose the ability to use certain objects such as combs and razors. They may forget what these objects are used for, forget that a task needs doing, lose interest in keeping clean, and as mentioned before, a loss of sense of time may make them believe that these tasks have been done.

Eating and drinking problems can be experienced. Not only do people with Alzheimer's disease experience difficulty in using utensils but their eating habits may change. Some people hoard foods, others start to eat everything in sight and others just eat one thing only.

Incontinence (wetting and soiling) often occurs with Alzheimer's disease. Urinary incontinence is most common but faecal incontinence may occur, especially towards the end of the illness.

Problems with personal relationships can occur with Alzheimer's disease. It is common for a person with Alzheimer's disease not to recognise his partner and to experience fear on waking up to what they think is a total stranger. Also people with Alzheimer's disease may experience reduced sexual demands and/or increased sexual demands.

5) Behavioural Changes

Alzheimer's disease causes a variety of behavioural changes such as agitation, aggression, following around, fits, hallucinations, hiding objects, repetitive questioning and wandering at night.

Agitation is when a person appears restless and irritable. They may pace up and down or fiddle with everything in sight.

Aggression can be verbal and physical. This can mean swearing and striking out. Aggression is a normal human response to certain situations but people with Alzheimer's disease display it more than usual.

Sometimes people with Alzheimer's disease follow their carer around, all day from one room to the next, depriving the carer of privacy and relaxation.

In some cases of Alzheimer's disease a person experiences a fit, which resembles epilepsy. This is caused by a burst of electrical activity arising from brain cells. This is a consequence of dementia. The fit may consist of a repetitive movement of the hand or arm or the person could become rigid, clench their teeth and jerks. Sometimes breathing can stop.

People with dementia can experience hallucinations, when they hear, smell or feel something that does not exist.

Dealing with Dementia

Alzheimer's disease can make people hide objects due to a fear that someone will steal them.

Asking questions over and over again is also a common aspect of Alzheimer's disease. Forgetting that they have already asked the question and received an answer may cause this.

Sleep disturbances can cause a person with Alzheimer's disease to wander at night. Wandering can also occur during the day. They may slip out of the house, wander off and get lost.

The above symptoms are not the only symptoms of Alzheimer's disease and a person with Alzheimer's disease does not necessarily experience all of them. In a study by EUROCARE [34], the spouses of twenty elderly people with Alzheimer's disease in fourteen countries in the European Union were interviewed. Murray and Schneider (1998) reported that carers found the following problems the most difficult to cope with:

1	Loss of language/communication	24%
2	Loss of memory	17%
3	Aggression	17%
4	Uncooperative/stubborn behaviour	16%
5	Need for constant supervision/entrapment	14%
6	Spouse's personal care needs	13%
7	Disorientation	11%
8	Apathy	6%
9	Restlessness	5%
10	Personality changes	5%

Because the illness is so devastating and global, affecting not only the person, but also the spouse and family, and the relationships between family members, the family must try to work together to help to improve the patient's quality of life. This is no easy task, as any family carer knows. There are no easy answers and sometimes super-human powers are required.

The Fédération Associations Alzheimer's Sud-Europe (FASE) has provided guidelines on how to promote the quality of life of people with Alzheimer's[8]. For example, it is recommended to help the person to maintain their personal hygiene for as long as possible. This can be aided by regularly encouraging them to take a warm bath or shower with stimulating, positive remarks, such as: "You are going to feel better"; "It's ready, go on, the water will get cold" and by putting a sign on the bathroom door, written or drawing. By making simple adaptations to the home environment and finding simpler ways for communicating, many activities of daily living can be supported.

Stages of development

The problems with Alzheimer's disease that have been described do not happen all at once. At first the difficulty with memory and loss of intellectual abilities may go unnoticed, as they are so slight. As the illness progresses, the symptoms become more noticeable and they start to interfere with everyday life. Experiences of confusion, changes of mood and language may be the first signs that there is a problem. Difficulties with daily living activities such as dressing, washing and going to the toilet eventually become so severe that the person becomes totally dependent on others. Alzheimer's Disease usually leads to death within ten years. The most common cause of death is pneumonia because, as the disease progresses the immune system worsens, and there is weight loss, which make the risk of throat and lung infections greater.

Conclusions

There are many different forms of dementia and each is associated with its own pattern of changes in the affected individual. The two most common forms, Alzheimer's disease and multi-infarct (or vascular) dementia, are often mis-diagnosed and get mixed together. It is important to try to understand the changes that occur in the person who is affected. Early, accurate diagnosis is the first essential of good dementia care.

KEY TERMS

Alzheimer's disease

Alzheimer's disease and related disorders (ADRD)

Creutzfeldt-Jakob disease (CJD)

Huntington's disease (Huntington's chorea)

Korsakoff's syndrome

Lewy-body disease

Multi-infarct dementia

Parkinson's disease

Pick's disease

Senile dementia

CHAPTER 2:   WHAT CAUSES ALZHEIMER'S DISEASE?

In this chapter we briefly discuss the changes in the brain and nervous system that are associated with Alzheimer's disease. In asking what causes Alzheimer's disease, it must be stated at the outset that we simply do not know. Hundreds of researchers are currently working on this question and, when it comes, the answer will be a major breakthrough. At present we have some clues about the cause(s) of the disease from investigations of the many changes that occur in the brains of people with Alzheimer's disease.

The most important changes used in confirming a diagnosis of Alzheimer's disease are referred to as plaques and tangles. At present this confirming diagnosis can only be done by post-mortem examination.

Plaques, Tangles and Beta-Amyloid Deposition

These changes occur in the neurones (nerve cells) in the brain. To understand these changes, a basic understanding of the structure of neurones is needed. Figure 2.1 shows the structure of a neurone.

The tree-like branches called dendrites receive chemical messages from other neurones. The messages then flow through the cell body, then the axon to the dendrites of other neurones.

The messages from one neurone can therefore be sent along the dendrites of many other neurones.

Figure 2.1: The important features of a neurone

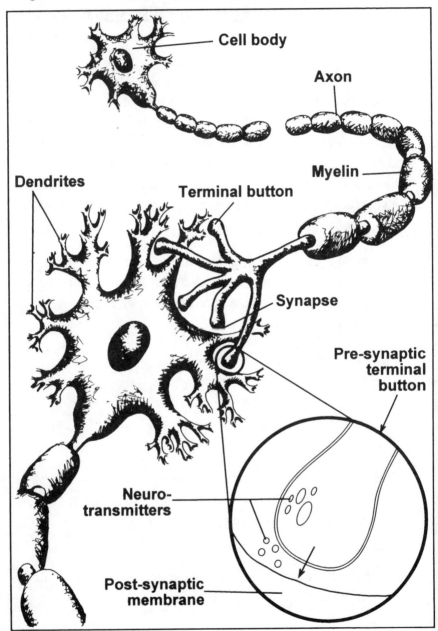

Plaques occur in the part of the brain where the axons are contained. Plaques contain a massive protein core of *beta-amyloid protein* that does not occur naturally in the brain. Plaques interfere with the messages being sent from neurone to neurone. At present, it is not known how or why these plaques are formed. However they are associated with the deposition of beta-amyloid protein. The mechanisms are probably rather complicated and there are many possible causal pathways.

The tangles occur in the cell body of brain neurones. They are bundles of long thread-like structures. These threads consist of helical filaments twisted around each other in pairs like a spiral. It is not known how or why the tangles are formed. Their main constituent is tau protein.

Plaques and neurofibrillary tangles also occur in the brains of elderly people without Alzheimer's disease. However they are much more frequent in the brains of people with Alzheimer's disease. Plaques and tangles are not equally present in all parts of the brain. They are most common in areas of the brain known as the hippocampus and the cerebral cortex.

The hippocampus has a vital role in memory and the cerebral cortex is the centre for various complex mental processes such as initiating voluntary actions, language and speech, perceiving the world, and finding one's way around unfamiliar environments. It has recently been observed that the remaining neurones in the hippocampus can sprout and form new connections with other neurones to replace those that have been lost.

Although plaques and tangles are associated with Alzheimer's disease, they are not necessarily the cause. Another more basic process may cause the formation of plaques and tangles and also cause Alzheimer's disease itself. It is likely that there is no single cause of Alzheimer's disease and the other conditions associated with dementia. In fact, there are likely to be many different causes for each one of the different conditions associated with dementia. In all probability the causes will be an interaction of genetic and environmental factors, including diet. At present, because we lack any direct knowledge of the causes, we lack the ability to produce a cure for dementia.

Neurotransmitters and Alzheimer's Disease

In addition to the core mechanisms of the disease process discussed above, there are also some more peripheral processes associated with the symptoms of dementia. When chemical messages pass from the axon of one neurone to the dendrites of others, they must pass over a small gap, known as a *synapse*, that separates the two (see Figure 2.1). When the neurone sending the message releases a chemical known as a *neurotransmitter* from the terminal buttons, the gap at the synapse is bridged. The neurone's receptors on the other side detect the presence of the neurotransmitter and the message is received.

Acetylcholine is a neurotransmitter that occurs in the brain. In people who do not have Alzheimer's disease, the amount of acetylcholine remains fairly constant. However people with Alzheimer's disease have a reduced amount of acetylcholine in their brains. It is thought that the loss of acetylcholine may result in the deterioration of memory and possibly cause other Alzheimer's symptoms.

The term "*cholinergic system*" is used to describe the system of neurones that uses acetylcholine. Like plaques and tangles, neurotransmitter levels can only be directly studied after death. However, once a brain is dead, chemical changes occur rapidly and so the neurotransmitters can only be studied very soon after death. It is for this reason that acetylcholine is rarely studied itself. Rather a substance called choline acetyltransferase (ChAT) is used as an indicator of the neurotransmitter as it remains quite stable in the brain for hours after death. ChAT is used by the neurones to make acetylcholine, so a lack of ChAT indicates a lack of acetylcholine.

Drugs that work on the cholinergic system are available today. These drugs appear to slow the progression of AD in the early stages. Because they work only at the level of reducing the symptoms, and do not produce a cure, the drugs are referred to as "symptomatic" rather than curative. Drugs used for treating dementia are discussed in Chapter 8. Before learning more about treatment, however, we need to understand how dementia is diagnosed.

Conclusions

In spite of a large amount of research, the causes of Alzheimer's disease and most other forms of dementia still remain a mystery. Alzheimer's disease is associated with the appearance of plaques, tangles and deposits of beta-amyloid in particular regions of the brain. The most popular theory of Alzheimer's disease is that it is caused by a breakdown in the cholinergic system of transmission between nerve cells. Drugs that work on this system appear to slow the progression of the disease. However research continues on the central causes of the neurodegeneration that occurs in all forms of dementia.

KEY TERMS

Acetylcholine

Amyloid

Cholinergic system

Neurotransmitter

Plaques

Tangles

CHAPTER 3:   ASSESSMENT AND DIAGNOSIS

Because we do not yet know the cause of the disease, and therefore don't really know what biological signs to look for, it is impossible to say with 100 percent accuracy that a living person has Alzheimer's disease. Only post mortem examination of brain tissue can identify the changes that are associated with the disease and confirm a provisional diagnosis. A reliable method for accurate diagnosis in the early stages of the disease that uses a biological marker is still being looked for. When such a method is discovered it will also be possible to develop effective methods of prevention and treatment. In the meantime it is necessary to rely upon psychological and neuropsychiatric tests in combination with brain imaging.

In order to make a preliminary diagnosis of Alzheimer's disease, an assessment of a patient's symptoms and mental abilities is made, normally by a family doctor, neurologist, gerontologist, psychiatrist, neuropsychologist or clinical psychologist. The doctor or psychologist will usually talk to the person thought to have Alzheimer's disease and also to someone who knows the person well from the patient's family.

Diagnosis

It is often difficult to be obtain a reliable, differential diagnosis of Alzheimer's disease. It is necessary to rule out the possibility that the experienced symptoms have a different and perhaps more easily treatable cause. Other illnesses, which can cause similar symptoms, must first be eliminated from, or added to the diagnosis:

Depression has some similar symptoms to Alzheimer's

disease including apathy, sleep disturbances and changes in eating habits. The main symptom of depression is a deeply sad mood. It is important to rule out depression as this can be treated with therapy or medication. People with dementia may also suffer from depression. It is important to identify depression in someone with dementia as treating the depression can help him or her to feel better. Having two or more illnesses at the same time is known as "co-morbidity". Dementia with depression is the most common form of co-morbidity when dementia is involved.

Hypothyroidism is an underactivity of the thyroid gland and it can produce dementia. It can be treated with replacement thyroid hormones.

Head injury resulting in a "sub-dural haematoma", a large blood clot between the skull and the membrane covering the brain, can be treated and cured surgically.

Hydrocephalus, a build-up of fluid in the brain, can be treated by inserting a tube to drain the fluid.

Vitamin deficiency, particularly of B group vitamins, and especially B12 after the age of 50 because of poor absorption. This can be treated.

Infections in the very old can produce an "acute confusional state". These can be treated with antibiotics.

Once these other illnesses have been ruled out, other forms of assessment are used to diagnose dementia. The CNEOPSA (Care Needs of Minority Ethnic Older Persons Suffering from Alzheimer Disease) project[15] noted that there are several professional groups who may make a diagnosis for dementia. These are psychogeriatricians, other psychiatrists, neurologists and community practice nurses.

One problem with this situation is that these professionals are likely to diagnose dementia in different ways using different and sometimes inconsistent criteria. We need standard diagnostic criteria that do not vary across health professionals. This should be able to produce a reliable diagnosis whichever health professional makes it. Accurate diagnosis is the first essential step towards optimum care.

Mini Mental State Examination

The *Mini Mental State Examination* or the "mini mental" as it is known for short, is a commonly used screening test for dementia. It takes approximately five minutes and involves performing a set of tasks. A score out of a maximum of thirty is given. Examples of items are:

What is the (year) (season) (date) (day) (month)?
Where are we: (state) (country) (town) (hospital) (floor)?
Spell "world" backwards
Write a sentence

The mini mental can be useful for evaluating people's mental abilities in the early stages of dementia. However there are certain drawbacks. The authors of the CNEOPSA project [15] point out that although the mini mental is frequently used, research clearly shows that this test is inappropriate for different ethnic groups. Some studies have adapted commonly used assessment scales such as the mini mental for different communities (e.g. Spanish and Hindi) and have found that not only is this difficult, but some questions have to be completely changed to make them culturally sensitive. There have been some attempts to develop assessment tools that are more culturally sensitive. For example the Abbreviated Barcelona Test (ABT) has been developed for Spanish speaking communities.

Research carried out at the University of Crete [20] revealed an interesting finding. In 57% patients identified as having possible dementia through the mini mental, a score greater than five was obtained on the Geriatric Depression Scale, indicating that they are potentially depressive. Despite the fact that people with dementia do suffer from depression, this highlights the importance of ruling out other illnesses. A possible explanation of this finding could be linked to culture. People with dementia in Crete are often kept indoors, hidden away from their essentially outdoor society. This may be a possible reason for the high depression scores in this population.

Regardless of its drawbacks, the mini mental is still a commonly employed screening test in European research. This is no doubt due to the fact that it is quick and easy to use and provides researchers with comparable data.

Global Deterioration Scale (GDS)
This scale is specifically designed to reflect the characteristics of Alzheimer's Disease. Reisberg, Ferris, De Leon and Crook developed it in 1982 in the USA. The GDS is a seven point rating instrument that helps stage the disease. Table 3.1 shows the seven points of the GDS.

Table 3.1:   The seven points of the Global Deterioration Scale

1	No subjective complaints of memory deficit. No memory deficit evident on clinical interview.
2	A subjective complaint of memory deficit, especially names and places of objects. No objective evidence of memory deficit.

3   Earliest clear-cut deficits. Poorer memory, poorer performance, loss of concentration. Objective evidence obtained with intensive interview.

4   Clear-cut deficit on careful clinical interview often accompanied by denial, flattened affect, and withdrawal.

5   Patient can no longer survive without some assistance. Unable to recall a major aspect of their current life, e.g. their address or telephone number, names of close family members, the name of the school or college they attended.

6   May occasionally forget the name of spouse (or other relative/friend) upon whom they are entirely dependent for survival Requires assistance with activities of daily living. Diurnal rhythm frequently disturbed. Personality and emotional changes occur.

7   All verbal abilities are lost over the course of this stage. The person is incontinent. Basic psychomotor skills (e.g. ability to walk) are lost with the progression of this stage.

Source: Summarised from Reisburg et al., 1982

As Table 3.1 shows, the first two stages are evident only as a mild cognitive impairment that cannot be detected without some sophisticated testing. Reisberg has shown that there is a significant correlation between the level of GDS and scores on the MMSE. Many new testing procedures are being developed to provide early diagnosis of mild cognitive impairment and ADRD. Many of these methods rely upon the measurement of changes in Activities of Daily Living (ADL), e.g. the Bayer Activities of Daily Living Scale (B-ADL) assesses changes in 25 activities according to the level of difficulty experienced along a 10-point scale. These activities include personal hygiene, observing important dates or events, taking part in a conversation, shopping, preparing food, and using domestic appliances (Hindmarch, Lehfeld, de Jongh & Erzigkeit, 1998).

Brain Scans

Brain scans (or brain imaging) are not used for every diagnosis. However, if a patient's symptoms are not typical or if a doctor suspects a brain tumour, then a brain scan is usually done. Scans improve the detection of ADRD but, as yet, remain imperfect as a diagnostic tool.

The CT scan or the CAT scan (Computerised Axial Tomography) takes pictures of slices of the brain using X-rays and a computer. It usually takes about 15-30 minutes to do.

MRI (Magnetic Resonance Imaging) also uses a computer to create pictures of slices of the brain. However X-rays are not used for MRI scans. Instead radio signals produced by the body in response to the effects of a very strong magnet contained within the scanner are used. More detail is shown with a MRI scan but the procedure takes longer and is more expensive.

SPECT (Single Photon Emission Computerised Tomography) looks at blood flow through the brain and also produces computer-generated pictures of slices of the brain.

More recently the use of computerised brain atlases has allowed many new possibilities. MR images are made into computerised images that can be compared with a computerised atlas of the brain. This method has been applied to the study of different forms of dementia to improve the determination of the location and size of lesions in the brain.

Obtaining and disclosing a diagnosis

A booklet about ethics has been produced by the European Alzheimer's Clearing House in English, Dutch, French, German, Italian and Greek [11]. This booklet discusses the issue of obtaining and disclosing a diagnosis. Often family members and friends wonder what is the use and value of diagnosis. They worry about telling their family member that an Alzheimer's disease diagnosis has been made. They are afraid of upsetting them and wonder what is the benefit of them knowing. In Denmark the law requires disclosure. There are in fact several benefits and disadvantages of obtaining and informing the affected person about a diagnosis.

Advantages of obtaining and disclosing a diagnosis:

+ A diagnosis can differentiate between treatable and non-treatable forms of dementia. In both cases it can contribute to the planning of treatment and care.

+ A diagnosis makes it possible to identify the cause of symptoms and problems. This may provide a sense of relief because disturbing behaviours can be attributed to a disease that is not under the person with dementia's control.

+ Arrangements for the future with regard to legal, financial and care issues can be made. This may help the carer to carry out the person's wishes and prevent wondering whether they are doing the right thing.

+ Early diagnosis means that treatment and interventions can be applied in order to alleviate suffering and contribute to well being. Research shows that the drugs on the market are more effective during the early stages of Alzheimer's Disease.

+ A diagnosis may open the door to sources of financial help.

Disadvantages of obtaining and disclosing a diagnosis:

- The fact that at present there is no cure may create a feeling hopelessness.

- The diagnostic procedure may be a burdensome and worrying time.

- There is a risk that a diagnosis of Alzheimer's disease may be made when in fact the person does not have Alzheimer's disease.

- A diagnosis of Alzheimer's disease may change the perception and expectations of family or friends. They may change their behaviour in such a way that the person is "reduced" to their diagnosis.

Disclosing a diagnosis depends on individual circumstances. The carer needs to decide how useful they think it is telling the person that they have Alzheimer's disease. Making a list of personalised benefits and disadvantages can be useful in making the final decision.

Professor dr. R. Heinrich at Ludwig Maximillians University in Munich, Germany led a task force working on the development of European recommendations for the General Practitioner on diagnosis and therapy of dementia (Heinrich, 1998). The task force observed that patients tend to see their doctors at different Reisburg stages in different countries, e.g. in Italy, Spain and Greece, at stages 2-3, but in Portugal as stage 4. The task force concluded that, while family doctors are the gatekeepers in treating people with dementia, their ability to do the right thing at the right time is limited. The task force suggested that change is needed to fight ignorance through the increase of knowledge of more effective and accurate methods of diagnosis and treatment.

Professor Robert Moulias of the Société Francaise de Gérontologie conducted a project on the role of expert centres (or outpatients' clinics) in early diagnosis and care of Alzheimer's disease[7]. The diagnosis of dementia is difficult especially in the early phase of the disease. However early diagnosis can permit a delay in the evolution of the disease (by the administration of drugs), avoid the development of a crisis situation, limit hospitalisation and institutional care, and lead to the planning of realistic therapeutic strategies for home care. Professor Moulias and his team designed a survey to find out how 32 expert centres in 15 western European countries manage their role of making early diagnosis. The results were analysed in terms of diagnostic procedures, diagnostic criteria, and care plans, follow up, and the operational aspects of expert centres. It was surprising how widespread was the consensus in almost all of the fields of outpatient care.

The diagnostic procedures comprised differential and etiological diagnosis of various types of dementia and associated diseases. Diagnosis required a multidisciplinary assessment on one, two or three visits to the centre. The group decided to recommend the use of DSM IV criteria. A competent skilled professional who is trained in old age psychology and knows how to administer psychometric tests must perform neuropsychological assessment. This assessment must include at least memory, language, praxis, gnosis, and executive functions.

The principal carer must be present at the assessment and must be involved in the planning of care. A home visit may be necessary. Assessment of the carer's "burden" is essential for dementia management even in the early stages.

The content of the assessment should be as follows:

- Knowledge of the full medical and personal history

- Physical examination (including complete neurological examination)

- Psychological examination (including associated troubles, such as sleep, behavioural and mood disorders)

- Standard biological examination (blood tests, liver and kidney functions, glycemia, TSH, folates, vitamin B12)

- Optional examination for HIV, syphilis, APOE

- Chest X-ray, ECG

- Basic cerebral imaging (CT or IRM)

- Optional functional imaging (research purposes)

- Other possible examinations include: Doppler, EEG, echocardiography, CSF

- A nutritional assessment is absolutely necessary

Expert outpatients' centres should provide patients and carers with broad care plans and not just prescribe drugs. The specialist team in the centre should be multidisciplinary, collaborate with other medical and social partners, be linked and integrated with all professions needed for the care of people with dementia. The expert centre cannot do or provide everything. It should work in a network with the GP, community nurse, social workers, home care assistants and help educate these key players.

The care plan should result from a comprehensive assessment of needs focusing on:

- Patient's problems: physical, psychiatric, functional, social, and psychological

- Carer's issues, including finance

- Assessment should focus on care in the home

The care plan should aim at improving the quality of life of the patient and the carer. It should include assessment of the present situation and also the likely future concerns. The group of expert centres in Professor Moulias' survey suggested that further consideration should be given to the following issues:

- Specialised dementia nurses overseeing and training home care assistants should be explored

- There should be a legal right to request assessment of a patient's health and social needs

- Carers should be given a legal right to request assessment of their needs

Follow up needs to be organised to make sure that the care plan is set up properly and working well. The plan can be re-adjusted in this light and following any new events. The prerequisites of successful follow-up are that all relevant actors both inside and outside the home must be informed of the details of the proposals and on the reasons why they were made. The family needs to be informed in even more detail. It is necessary to have an agreed appropriation of tasks and responsibilities by all actors involved in the care. In making a decision to transfer the patient to residential care, the expert centre should protect the interests of the patient and her/his family, advise the family, inform the patient and prepare them for the change. To improve follow-up, we need a tool that is sensitive to the quality of life of the patient and the principal carer, a tool to measure the quality of co-ordination of care, and a tool to alert the care team and signal crisis.

The operation of expert centres should be associated with competencies in geriatrics, psychiatry, or better still, geriatric psychiatry, psychology and psychometrics, social advice, gerontological skills. The centre must have access to neurological advice, and all other medical and paramedical services (e.g. occupational therapy, physiotherapy) according to the needs of the patient and carer. The centre needs to be integrated into a large health centre or geriatric service of a hospital.

New treatments of dementia and proper development of outpatient care entail extra expenses.

However this may be counterbalanced by reduced hospitalisations and placements in institutions. The extra expense is also justified, as any other health expenditure, by a significant improvement in the quality of life of outpatients and their families.

Co-operation between European expert centres represents a major tool for making progress in dementia care. Professor Moulias' study group decided to continue their co-operation as a European Task Force on the outpatient care of dementia and for a better quality of life for patients and carers.

Conclusions

Present methods of diagnosis require the elimination of other diseases and the administration of paper-and-pencil tests such as the mini mental and also brain scans. Standards of diagnosis vary greatly between districts, regions and countries across Europe. Optimum methods need to be agreed to ensure that early diagnosis is possible in the most reliable and standardised way. More training of doctors and specialists on the diagnosis and care of dementia is needed throughout

Europe to increase the efficiency of diagnosis and quality of care. Expert outpatients' centres play a major role in early diagnosis and the development and follow up of care plans. There is a need for an expert centre in every district and region.

KEY TERMS

Activities of Daily Living (ADL)

Brain scan

Co-morbidity

DSM IV criteria

Expert centre

Global deterioration scale (GDS)

Mini Mental State Examination (or mini mental)

CHAPTER 4: PREVALENCE OF DEMENTIA

Current prevalence

How many men and women in Europe have dementia at the present time? The EURODEM Prevalence Research Group has produced the most comprehensive figures on the prevalence of dementia and AD in Europe. This collaborative effort of 12 centres co-ordinated by Professor A. Hofman and Dr L.J. Launer at the Department of Epidemiology and Biostatistics, Erasmus University Medical School, Rotterdam, the Netherlands[14]. The 12 centres are spread across Europe from Finland in the north to Italy and Spain in the south. The information collated from 13 population-based samples by the 12 centres can be assumed to be representative of the general European population. This information is given in Figure 4.1.

These data from the EURODEM group suggest that:

◆ Most (70%) cases are diagnosed as Alzheimer's Disease.

◆ After the age of 80, the number of women with dementia, particularly AD, is higher than the number of men with dementia.

◆ Currently approximately 1,260,000 men and 2,430,000 women 65 years of age and over living in the European Union suffer from dementia.

Current incidence

The EURODEM Prevalence Research Group also provided figures on incidence, the number of new cases per 1000 people in one year. The estimates suggest that there are 228,000 and

Figure 4.1:   The prevalence of dementia, Alzheimer's disease and vascular dementia

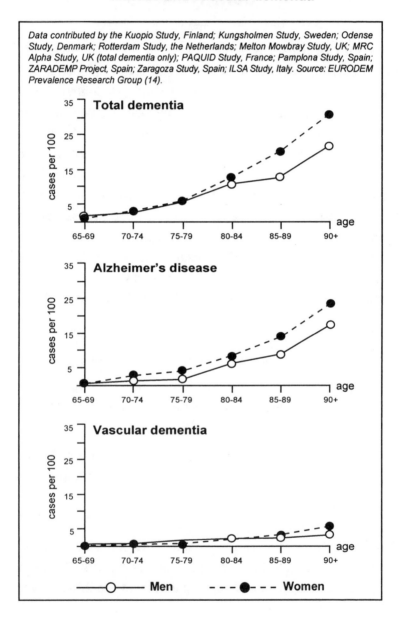

Data contributed by the Kuopio Study, Finland; Kungsholmen Study, Sweden; Odense Study, Denmark; Rotterdam Study, the Netherlands; Melton Mowbray Study, UK; MRC Alpha Study, UK (total dementia only); PAQUID Study, France; Pamplona Study, Spain; ZARADEMP Project, Spain; Zaragoza Study, Spain; ILSA Study, Italy. Source: EURODEM Prevalence Research Group (14).

596,000 new cases of dementia developing each year among European men and women respectively. As was the case with prevalence figures, even higher figures would be obtained if very mild cases of dementia were also included.

Prognosis

The EURODEM study also gave figures on *prognosis*, what happens to men and women with the disease compared to those without the disease. This was assessed in terms of the numbers of men and women living in institutions and in terms of death rates. The Rotterdam study showed that at 65 years of age, and at 85 years and over, men and women with dementia are over 30 times more likely to live in an institution than people who do not have dementia. At 65, men with dementia are three times more likely than women with dementia to live in an institution. At 85, men and women are equally likely to be living in an institution.

In terms of death rates:

◆ Individuals with dementia are 2.4 times more likely to die than individuals without dementia.

◆ Men with dementia are 1.7 times more likely to die from dementia than women with dementia.

◆ After five years of follow-up of individuals 85 years and older

-16% of men with dementia had survived, compared to 44% of men without dementia

-27% of women with dementia had survived, compared to 52% of women without dementia.

Future prevalence and incidence

For a lot of different reasons, people today are living longer than ever before. As the population becomes older and "greyer" over the next few decades, the incidence and prevalence of dementia is going to increase dramatically. The prevalence of dementia is expected to increase from the current figure of around 4.0 million people to at least 5.3 million in 2010, an increase of 33% (Wimo, 1998). In later decades the increases will continue still further, possibly levelling off at around 8-10 million people by the middle of the 21st century. Unless, of course, the cause(s) of ADRD can be discovered and effective treatments developed.

The increase in prevalence of dementia in the European is going to have many consequences for society. The greatest share of the responsibility for care is taken by the family and, in particular, by wives and daughters. As dementia cases increase, average family size is expected to decrease. Women today normally divide their time between paid employment and family responsibilities and when dementia strikes there is usually a drop in family income. This reduction in household income compounds the difficulties of caring for the family member who has been struck by dementia. It is going to get even tougher on carers in future unless the level of support given by social and health care is significantly raised. We return to the issues of informal care and the policy implications of demographic changes in Part Two.

Risk factors for dementia

Risk factors are biological, environmental or behavioural factors that increase the chances of illness striking. As research progresses, more risk factors are discovered while other candidates, previously considered as possibilities, are eliminated. The list of agreed risk factors is always much shorter than the list of possible risk factors. The four most commonly mentioned risk factors for dementia are:

◆   Age: the greater the age, the higher the risk (see Figure 7.1)

- Gender: women are at about twice the risk of men (see Figure 7.1)

- Education: the lower the level of formal education, the greater the risk, especially for women

- Apolipoprotein: the presence of the Apolipoprotein E-4 allele (APOE*4) increases the risk

  Source: Launer et al. 1999

Other risk factors include smoking and strokes. When two or more factors are present together, e.g. the APOE*4 allele and strokes, or the APOE*4 allele and arteriosclerosis, the risks may multiply rather than add.

Research at Erasmus University in Rotterdam by Kalmijn (1997) suggests the potential importance of diet and metabolic factors, previously rather neglected. Subject to confirmation in further research, the following factors may also increase risk:
- High amounts of linoleic acid
- High dietary fat, especially saturated fat, and cholesterol
- Low consumption of fish
- Homocysteine (an amino acid reduced by eating folates)
- Cortisol (an adrenal steroid)

Other factors that appear to increase risk include:
- Diabetes mellitus (both clinical and pre-clinical stages)
- Cardiovascular diseases (e.g. artherosclerosis, especially in people who have the APOE*4 allele; Ott, 1997)

On the other hand, high amounts of dehydroepiandrosterone sulphate (DHEAS; another adrenal steroid) may decrease the risk (Kalmijn, 1997).

These recent scientific studies show that diet has a strong influence on the health, especially on the kinds of diseases we may suffer late in life. As is the case for the other health scourges of cancer and cardiovascular disease, eating a healthy diet that is low in saturated fat could also protect against dementia. Recently, it has been suggested that a high cholesterol diet may cause Alzheimer's disease in Western society (Holden, 1999). Some recent evidence suggests that similar processes related to genetic susceptibility may cause arteriosclerosis and dementia (Slooter, 1998).

Other factors that may possibly increase the risk of dementia are exposure to:

◆ Aluminium
◆ Lead
◆ Solvents
◆ Pesticides
◆ Electromagnetic field

However, the above factors remain highly controversial and the evidence is inconsistent.

Conclusions

Hopefully, we will know the causes of Alzheimer's disease and the other forms of dementia in the near future. In the meantime, while researchers look for the causes, the best policy is to live as healthy a life as possible by avoiding smoking, foods containing large amounts of saturated fats and potential environmental hazards. We already know that living a healthy lifestyle and eating a healthy diet will lower the risk of cancer, heart disease, and strokes. Quite possibly healthy living decreases the risk of dementia as well. More epidemiological and medical studies are needed to determine the causes of the different kinds of dementia. Then we will be able to seek ways to prevent it altogether. Until then, we must improve public and professional understanding of dementia and allow those who suffer it the best possible care and quality of life.

KEY TERMS

Allele

Apolipoprotein

Incidence

Prevalence

Prognosis

Risk factor

Part Two:

Recent European Research

CHAPTER 5: INFORMAL CARE

In Part One we have seen that dementia is already highly prevalent and becoming increasingly so. Lacking a complete understanding of its principle causes, we have no methods of long-lasting treatment or prevention. It is therefore important to study the implications of dementia for families, services and social policy. In this way, we can learn as a society how best to deal with dementia. In Part Two we review recent European studies of dementia care, informal and formal, communication and information, treatments and interventions, equity, policy and economic issues and targets for the future.

Services in the public sector are already busily occupied and there may need to be increasing reliance in future on private, insurance-based systems of care. The provision of residential care and nursing homes varies between the European Union member states, and most do not have sufficient places to cater for their citizens with dementia. In at least 80 percent of cases, the patients' families are the principal carers for people with ADRD. Care provided by patients' families, neighbours or friends is referred to as "informal care". Zarit et al (1985) referred to informal carers as the "hidden victims" of dementia.

All families, and families with low incomes in particular, are likely to find themselves in a difficult situation when a family-member becomes ill with Alzheimer's or another form of dementia. Even if they can afford it and could manage to arrange it, residential care is not the option of choice for the great majority of families and so an increasing number of families will be relying on their own support mechanisms to care for their relatives with dementia (see Box 5.1). Terminology varies from country to country and the terms "carer" and "caregiver" are both used and have the same meaning. In this book we use the term "informal carer" for family members, friends or neighbours who provide care for a person with dementia.

Box 5.1:   **Mr Brown who cares for his mother**

Mr Brown is in his late 50s and has been caring for his elderly mother for four years, since she developed Alzheimer's Disease. Mr Brown has never been married and has lived with his mother all his life. After the death of his father, many years ago, Mr Brown bought a large house in the outskirts of London. He moved from the family home taking his sister and mother with him. Mr Brown's mother suffered a nervous breakdown following the death of her husband, and Mr Brown and his sister considered that their mother was not able to look after herself. Mr Brown thinks the reason he has never married is due to his mother is unable to look after herself.

Since caring for his mother, Mr Brown has been forced to give up his job as she is unable to be left alone, and she refuses to go to day care or to be cared for by most sitters. In addition to this, Mr Brown's mother constantly demands attention, requires constant entertainment, goes to bed very late, and wakes up and wanders throughout the night. Mr Brown is exhausted and feels that he has lost his 'life'. He cannot go out alone at any time during the day or night, apart from one evening a week when a sitter comes to care for his mother (after some persuasion). This, however, has its problems as the sitter will only stay until 10.30pm which limits socialising time to two hours which is not even enough time to go to the cinema. At home, Mr Brown cannot concentrate on anything that he enjoys or needs to attend to as his mother constantly "badgers him like a child", saying that she is bored.

Mr Brown resents his caring role as he has lost most of his friends and his job as a result of it. Having said that, however, Mr Brown loves his mother very much and seems to be a very caring and patient man. He won't even consider residential care as he says that 'being put in a home' has always been his mother's biggest fear.

The demands placed on informal carers can be formidable. Professor Klein points out that depression, aggression, violence, helplessness and burnout are some of the consequences for people involved in ADRD care[29]. Of course, not all carers experience these consequences. Some cope extremely well. However the very nature of ADRD is bound to pose some degree of challenge to any carer during its course. There is therefore a need to consider as a society how the affected families can best be supported as they learn to deal with AD and other forms of dementia. The well being of patients and families is therefore a primary concern.

Research on the well being of carers

There is a need to gain more understanding of the factors that influence the well being of informal carers who consist of families and friends, the majority of whom are female. In particular, the influence of economic, social and psychological factors associated with informal care warrants in-depth study. Carers frequently have poorer physical and psychological health than control samples. Behavioural disturbances in particular are strongly associated with carer stress. It is also known that stress is a strong predictor of admission to residential care at 6- or 12-month follow-up (Jerrom et al, 1993). Research on carers' well being can inform the development of interventions, programmes and policies intended to increase the coping resources of carers, which, in turn, should benefit people with dementia.

In this section we review the results of three studies conducted within the EC Alzheimer's programme concerned with the informal carer. Coincidentally all three studies were led by research groups based in London (Middlesex University, The Institute of Psychiatry, and the London School of Economics). Firstly, it is necessary to discuss terminology, language and culture, and how these affect the perception of the carer's role.

Much of this work on developing support for carers uses the concept of "carer burden". This term is controversial because it places a negative connotation on the challenges and opportunities that are presented by carers in dealing with dementia. Justine Schneider and Joanna Murray (1998) [34] describe carer burden in the following way:

> *Caring is part of many human relationships. In personal relationships it implies protection, supervision, feeling concern, and taking charge of. For the most part it is reciprocal, there is 'give and take'. But when one partner becomes dependent upon the other, there is no longer a balance between giving and taking, and new dynamics enter the relationship. This imbalance has been called 'burden'.*

Schneider and Murray, however, draw attention to the different associations of the word "burden" in different European languages. In English, "burden" has negative connotations, implying that the person receiving care is a nuisance, tiresome and costly to support. When Schneider and Murray translated the word "burden" into some other European languages, the direct translation seemed too negative (e.g. "burda" in Swedish and "fardo" in Portuguese). Less negative translations had associations of responsibility (e.g. "charges" in French; "carga" in Spanish and "cargo" in Italian') but even here the terms take away the sufferers' humanity and imply a more object-like status rather than a person.

A more neutral and less offensive term is "carer stress". This term avoids the derogatory reference to the person with ADRD as a burden. It implies only that the carer may experience stress to varying degrees. The ability to cope with stresses will depend on the resources that are available to the individual carer from a mixture of personal, family and external sources (Lazarus & Folkman, 1980; Pearlin et al, 1990).

The different nuances in meaning that occur as we attempt to translate words and ideas into different languages draw attention to the cultural differences that exist more generally in how caring for a person with dementia is seen in different societies. In some cultures caring for a family member or friend is seen as a great effort and beyond the call of duty, whereas other cultures see caring as a normal part of family life. Another cultural difference occurs in relation to the concept of "informal care." In a Swedish study investigating support for carers of people with ADRD, no family carers in the study could be deemed "informal carers"[27]. This was a reflection of the Swedish health and social care system and culture where there is an expectation that the state has a principle role in providing care. The informal carers in the study were therefore simply family members who provided a more limited level of support, in the form of visits and telephone contact.

Cultural differences towards caring also exist within countries. In Italy and Portugal major differences exist between the north and south owing to immigration factors and different levels of traditional family support. Also professional help, social support and available resources are generally far from uniform across countries, regions and districts[17].

Whatever the culture, caring for a person with ADRD requires considerable physical and psychological effort and can put a strain on finances. It can be a very demanding and stressful experience caring for a loved one who is going through the difficult changes that dementia brings, as hearing what carers say on this subject can leave little doubt:

> *I wish that this was not happening.*
> *I feel torn apart to see my person change like this.*
> *I felt irritable, angry, puzzled, saddened, depressed by the things s/he does.*
> *The loss of my person as s/he used to be leaves me feeling rattled, vulnerable, insecure, cheated, bitter.*
> *All this 'talking positive' about dementia is all very well for professional but they should try living with it, day in day out, and see how positive they feel then.*
>
> *Source: Schweitzer, P. (Ed.). (1998). Reminiscence in Dementia Care. London: Age Exchange, p 51*

The Middlesex /EACH study

A study was carried out by the authors on carer well being in association with the European Alzheimer's Clearing House (EACH)[11]. The methods and theory behind the study were based on similar studies on family coping conducted in Belgium by Professor Franz Baro and colleagues (Baro et al, 1996). The overall approach of the EACH work on carer support is based on the interactive model of the stress proposed by Pearlin et al (1990). The study is described in more detail in a separate publication (Marks, Pitt, Thomas, and Sykes, 1999).

A sample of 235 informal carers living in England, primarily in London and the Southeast, volunteered to be interviewed about their experiences. The participants were contacted via local branches of the Alzheimer's Disease Society and other carers' associations. As self-selected volunteers, however, they cannot be considered as representative of all ADRD carers. There were 148 women and 87 men in the sample. One hundred and forty were spouses, 76 were daughters or sons, 9 were siblings, 5 other relatives, and 5 were friends. The sample cared for people with a mixture of different kinds of dementia: 119 had a diagnosis of Alzheimer's disease; 28 had multi-infarct dementia; 78 were diagnosed with an unspecified form of dementia; and 10 did not know their diagnosis.

We analysed a range of factors thought to be contributing to the carers' stress levels. Factors investigated included carer's education, strength of religious beliefs, family disagreements, social support, amount of key services used, household income, time since the onset of the dementia, disability levels, recent fatigue and a psychological concept known as Sense of Coherence (SOC; see Box 5.2).

The study obtained some interesting findings. The aspects of ADRD that carers reported that they found most problematic were:

1   Disruption of their personal and social life

2   Appears anxious/agitated/frustrated

3   Not being able to leave person with dementia alone

4   Inability to hold a sensible conversation and forgetting things that have happened.

5   Unsteadiness of person with dementia on feet

6   Restless - on the move

7   Sudden mood changes and not being safe if outside the house alone

8   Incontinence (wetting)

9   Inability to do useful things

10 Person with dementia falling and sleep disturbances at night including wandering.

Box 5.2:   **Sense of Coherence (SOC)**

Aaron Antonovsky developed the SOC concept in 1987. Sense of coherence refers to the sense that certain areas of life matter, that they are challenges worthy of time and effort. According to Antonovsky (1987) sense of coherence is a "*global orientation that expresses the extent to which one has a pervasive, enduring though dynamic feeling of confidence that:*

(1)   the stimuli deriving from one's internal and external environments in the course of living are structured, predictable, and explicable;

(2)   the resources are available to one to meet the demands posed by these stimuli; and

(3)   these demands are challenges, worthy of investment and engagement."

These three components are otherwise known as comprehensibility, manageability, and meaningfulness.

People have different levels of SOC. Antonovsky suggested that having a strong sense of coherence could protect a person from breakdown in the face of highly stressful life situations. We found that a strong sense of coherence was associated with a lower level of stress (see Box 5.3). This observation confirms in a larger sample the earlier research conducted in Belgium by Professor Franz Baro at the Katholieke Universiteit in Leuven. Further studies are being conducted in eight different countries.

Box 5.3: **Mr White who has a high sense of coherence**

Mr White cares for his father who lives five minutes away. His father has Alzheimer's Disease and heart disease. He has also had cancer. Mr White's father can be quite challenging. For example, he is restless, continuously on the move, he is incontinent, always asking questions and he needs help with his meals. Mr White promised his father that he would not allow him to go into residential care. Therefore there is a purpose for Mr White in caring for his father. For one thing he is carrying out a promise.

Mr White is a religious man, married with two children. He manages to see his father every day. He is very well organised. He co-ordinates care rotas when he is unable to visit his father. He greatly acknowledges certain individuals who help him care for his father. Mr White is a professional and his job allows him to work around his father's needs. Mr White is able to mange his father's care. He is the type of person who comprehends his feelings and in general sees the situations that he finds himself in, in the right proportion. Rather than get upset and worried about his father, he views himself as the 'administrator of his care'. Mr White filled out a questionnaire to measure his sense of coherence and obtained a high score.

The European Alzheimer's Clearing House aims to develop support programmes intended to increase the level of SOC in family carers[11]. In this way it is hoped that the carers' coping mechanisms and the patients' informal care can be improved. Antonovsky himself believed that SOC was a stable trait that in general did not change during adulthood. Professor Baro and the EACH team are challenging this assumption and it is certainly worthwhile to do so. Whether or not carers' can increase their sense of coherence through supportive intervention remains an open question and will require careful evaluation.

The information collected in the Middlesex/EACH interview survey[11] suggested other correlates of carer stress:

1   Carer's fatigue in the last month

2   The disability level of the person being cared for (as indicated by the number of activities of daily living that were affected)

3   Family disagreements (see Box 5.4)

4   The education level of the person with ADRD

Factors that appeared unrelated to carer stress or 'burden' were:

1   Key services used (home care assistance, day care and other)

2   Social support

3   Household income

Box 5.4:   **Mrs Jackson who cares for her mother**

Mrs Jackson is a married woman in her late 40s. She cares for her mother who has Alzheimer's Disease. She moved her mother in with her when her father died 5 years ago. Mrs Jackson has a full-time job and two teenaged children. Her mother cannot be left alone, she demands attention, and she follows Mrs Jackson around constantly. She goes to a day care centre 5 days a week.

Mrs Jackson's brother has cared for their mother at weekends for a while. However, this has stopped since she discovered that he had been putting their mother into respite care while he should have been caring for her at home. Mrs Jackson found that her mother was disturbed and disorientated when she returned home on Sunday evenings each week. She found that it was taking until the middle of the week for her mother's behaviour to settle down. After having found out that her mother had been sent to a residential home at weekends, she refused to allow her brother to care for her any more, which led to conflicts and stress. Mrs Jackson feels that she needs his help desperately, but that he is not prepared to give up any of his time to take care of their mother. The care that he has been giving has caused more problems in the long run.

Her children, on the other hand, are very helpful and they offer to sit with their grandmother. However, she feels that this is unfair on her children as they are young and need their freedom. She feels that the responsibility lies with her and her brother. However, her brother is not prepared to give his time. Mrs Jackson resents this, as she cannot spend valuable time with her children at the weekends any more.

These findings are interesting and, in part, a little surprising. It was found that informal carers who reported more stress were:

◆ More fatigued over the last four weeks

◆ Looking after someone with more severe dementia

◆ Had a low sense of coherence

◆ Had more disagreements with the rest of the family

◆ Caring for a person with dementia who had received **more** education.

Surprisingly, the amount of social support carers received, the amount of key services used and a carer's household income were **not** factors that correlated significantly with carer stress. Although carers who had a higher education level themselves were receiving more services, the services being received did not appear to correlate with their need for those services as measured by the carers' stress scores.

What seems surprising is the fact that the amounts of services and social support received do not seem to be related with the everyday stress levels of the carers. Other factors such as the carer's fatigue over the last month, the disability level of the person being cared for, family disagreements, the person with dementia's education, seem to be having more influence on carer stress or burden. Helpful and vital though they are, it appears that services and social supports are unrelated to the felt severity of carer stress.

It might be expected that carers with the highest stress levels would be receiving more help and support and those with the lowest stress levels would be receiving less help and support i.e. that there would be a positive association between carer stress and services received. However, across this sample, there was no evidence of such a relationship - the amount of help and support a carer was receiving was unrelated to their stress levels. The current support systems, both professional and informal, appear to be unrelated to the carers' immediate needs.

These findings help us to gain some perspective on the formidable task faced by the dementia carer. They have a number of implications. They suggest that even the limited supports that are available are failing to "hit the target". While a few hours in a day care centre, and a visit or a chat on the telephone with a friend or relative may well bring some temporary relief or social contact, **dealing with dementia is a 24 hours a day, 365 days of the year responsibility**. One of the best-known carer manuals is in fact entitled the "Thirty Six Hour Day" (Mace et al, 1985). The available resources to support a carer come and go and, although they may well be a blessed relief while they last, they are having a transient effect, a short-lived sharing of a responsibility that has little impact on the overall stress level experienced by the full-time carer.

Another important finding relates to education: we found that the higher the education level of the person with ADRD, the greater the stress on the carer. This also has interesting implications. What follows is speculative, based on common sense understandings and assumptions rather than technical or scientific data. One possibility is that people with ADRD may experience the changes to their mental worlds in three related ways. Firstly is the overall loss of control over thoughts and actions. Secondly is the narrowing of the range of experience and activities, as the loss of control becomes more serious. Thirdly is the lack of stimulation as the everyday activities that are available reduce in number, e.g. watching television, visits to a day care centre. These available activities may not cater very well for the life-long interests of highly educated people. They may struggle to maintain activities that are impossible within the confusing experience of thoughts and perceptions that dementia brings (e.g. reading). The lack of stimulation brought by well-intentioned but more general communal activities is bound to lead to frustration, depression and behavioural problems.

The EUROCARE project

The second project concerned with informal carers was conducted by the EUROCARE research collaboration. Justine Schneider, Joanna Murray, Sube Banerjee and Anthony Mann of the Sections of Epidemiology and Old Age Psychiatry at the Institute of Psychiatry, University of London, led this project. The EUROCARE project[34] studied the experiences of spouses caring for people with dementia. The sample consisted of 20 carers from each of 14 EU Member States (all except Germany). The study explored the impact of coping with dementia, material assistance and social support in relation to measures of carer 'burden' and mental health. Pearlin's (1990) model guided the analysis of data from the EUROCARE study.

The characteristics of the samples across the 14 countries showed a number of significant differences. Unfortunately the small sizes and lack of representativeness of the national samples means that conclusions about national differences are unreliable. However the data for the sample of 280 carers as a whole provided some interesting and meaningful findings. The results showed that only 30% belonged to any kind of support group and only about a half received assistance from family and friends. On average family members helped them for 5.33 hours per week, although 52% received none. The analysis of the data for the 280 carers suggested that membership of support groups, total number of hours of home care received, and total amount of supporting informal care received from family and friends were showing no significant relationships with the carers' stress levels. These data confirm the UK Middlesex/EACH findings in a large transnational sample that **neither formal support nor social support is significantly related to carers' stress experience**. In fact the levels of formal help at home with personal care, nursing or domestic tasks was quite modest, with only 48% of couples receiving any at all. However overnight care or day care was being used at some point by a considerable proportion of people except in Ireland, Portugal, Greece, Holland and Spain.

Another interesting finding resulted from a question about how **satisfied** the carers were with their financial situation. Murray and Schneider reported that financial dissatisfaction was associated with higher "burden" scores. Sixty-one percent stated that they had additional expenses because of their spouse's dementia, although far fewer received any financial assistance. Apparently it is not the actual amount of money that a carer has available, but how **satisfied** they are with this amount that contributes to their stress levels. For example one carer might have a certain amount a year available and feel he can manage to care for his wife with this amount and maintain their normal standard of living. However another carer might receive the same amount and be constantly worried about money. This could be because they had previously been used to different living standards. Perhaps there were now extra living costs resulting from new needs, e.g. perhaps her husband with dementia now required services such as a barber or chiropodist at home that she has to pay for, or they might be used to a more expensive diet, and there could be all sorts of other reasons. How well off a person **feels** is probably as important as their actual income, not only among informal carers, but also in people in general.

Passive behavioural problems were more 'burdensome' than active behavioural problems. Also older carers felt less burdened. The perceived 'burden' of care was greater when other people were seen by the carer to react negatively to the dementia sufferer. Schneider and Murray[34] conclude that the EUROCARE study has implications for health and social policy, suggesting the need for more public education to improve the public image of dementia and also the situation of informal carers. We return to these issues in Chapter 10.

The "socio-economic burden" of informal care

The third study of the well being of informal carers was conducted by Franco Sassi and David McDaid at the London School of Economics[33]. This study aimed to measure aspects of the "burden" borne by informal carers of people with AD living in the community in Italy, Sweden and the United Kingdom and to determine whether this was affected by:

- ◆ Gender, age, social class, income and education of carers
- ◆ Availability and type of support programmes for carers
- ◆ Availability and access to formal health and social services for people with AD
- ◆ Clinical condition of the person with AD

The main hypothesis was that, controlling for other factors, the use of formal services would "reduce the burden of informal care".

The study began by attempting to recruit carers through General Practitioners (GPs) in all three countries using the same methodology of a telephone interview. However ethical issues, cultural differences and referral differences meant that the original intentions could not be carried out. Multiple and complex procedures for recruiting carers were found necessary which varied between countries. The demographic characteristics of the three national samples showed many highly significant differences making national comparisons impossible. However, the methodological problems with the study forced the authors to conclude that: "the type of study design could not provide insights on the question of whether and to what extent the use of formal services may help reducing the burden of formal care" (p. 201). The obtained results went in exactly the opposite direction to that predicted and carers reporting higher "burden" were found to be using more services. This is exactly the result one would expect if services were being targeted accurately at those most in need.

Lessons to be learned from the three studies on carer stress
The above three studies expose a number of problems with research on carers. Certainly none of the studies was perfect. There are valuable lessons that can be learned about the design and methodology of future studies:

There is a need for samples to be representative of carers in the general population, not simply opportunistic or convenience samples of volunteers obtained using non-random methods of selection. All three studies suffered from recruitment problems and consequently took all available participants with loose (or no) explicit criteria for inclusion or exclusion and little control over demographic or personal characteristics.

There is a need for sample sizes to be large enough to make statistical testing of the results reliable and meaningful. Two of the three studies used national sample sizes that were too small to make any reliable national comparisons although, in theory, it had been intended to investigate national differences.

There is a need for longitudinal research on carer well being and its psychological, social, and economic determinants. Only in controlled **prospective designs** will it be possible to test causal hypotheses about the determinants of carer stress. All three studies used cross-sectional designs that permit correlational rather than causal hypothesis testing. To be fair to the investigators, all were operating under tight time constraints with only one or two years to complete the studies. This meant that for good practical reasons the research had to use a **cross-sectional survey**.

Similarly, if we are to understand how services affect carer well being, it will be necessary in the future to conduct properly controlled longitudinal evaluations. Such studies are very rare and there have been hardly any studies of this kind in Europe.

There is an urgent need to investigate not only the effect of services on the well being of informal carers, but on the well being of people with dementia themselves. None of the above three studies attempted to evaluate directly the well being of dementia sufferers. This is a challenging aspect of dementia research because making judgements about the state of mind of a person with dementia is highly problematic and requires special communication skills. This is no reason why such communication should not be attempted. Too often, the focus is exclusively on the carer rather than on the person they are caring for, and the relationship between the two. We discuss the issue of communication in Chapter 7.

The studies reviewed above contain some flaws in methodology that should be avoided in future studies investigating the impact of services or interventions. As the LSE authors themselves acknowledge, the only way to test a causal hypothesis that "formal services reduce burden" is to do a longitudinal study comparing two matched or randomly allocated groups of carers, one group who receives the services and another group who does not receive the services. A design of the latter type is seen in the EDIF project [31] reviewed in Chapter 6. However, in spite of the excellent use of randomisation in the latter study, the sample sizes were too small to permit sufficient statistical power to test the impact of the intervention.

Because of the methodological problems with the studies, the conclusions drawn remain little more than speculations that require further research before any really solid answers can be given. Methodological differences between studies often help explain the conflicting results. What remains clear is that every individual has a very unique and special character or personality with a particular life history of experiences, habits, preferences and interests. What is a stressful "burden" to one person may be an uplifting challenge to another. There are undoubtedly rewarding aspects of caring for a person with dementia. There are positive rewards from selfless actions including the realisation of the value of human existence and the strengthening of the bonds that can occur between family members.

Some carers spontaneously adopt a person-centered approach to care without realising it. Other carers need a little more guidance. It has become incorporated into training programmes for both informal and formal carers and into many care manuals.

Training for informal carers

Families are the major provider of care to people with dementia and this group are making a huge contribution to society that is often unrecognised. By looking after their family members or friends, informal carers are reducing the costs of residential care. Training of informal carers therefore should be beneficial to the carer, the person they are caring for, and to society as a whole.

Dr Jacques Selmes, a member of EACH[11], points out that one of the advantages of home care is that mental stimulation is more interesting and suitable to the person's needs because the affected person's interests are better understood by family members than would generally be the case in an institution. However if people feel they are unable to care for family and friends, institutionalised care needs to be of a sufficiently high standard that family members do not to feel guilty about their decision to have their loved one placed in an institution.

The "H.O.M.E." - Helping Older people with dementia be Maintained at home through Education and training - Project was founded on the principle that improving carer support should be actively promoted[27]. The Northern Ireland partner of H.O.M.E. reviewed the literature on the impact of training and education on carers. All writers on this subject appeared to be in agreement that it is important to enable family carers to:

♦ Maintain a positive relationship with the patient
♦ Prevent institutionalisation
♦ Improve the quality of life for patients and carers
♦ Recognise the carer as an expert
♦ Reduce carer stress regarding care giving

However, until the H.O.M.E. project itself, there was no clear evidence that carer training actually achieves any of these objectives. The H.O.M.E. project therefore set out to identify the support, information and skill needs of carers (informal and formal) in Northern Ireland, Ireland, Portugal and Sweden. Carers actively took part in this process by helping to shape and influence the content of training. The training courses were then evaluated.

The H.O.M.E. project found that informal carers generally believed that training would be useful in the early stages of their career as a carer. This was particularly evident in Northern Ireland where most of the carers reported *higher* stress scores **after** attending the training courses. However the person with the shortest length of time in caring had a *decreased* stress score after the training which is what the trainers expected. One reason the carers' stress scores were higher after the training could be that the carers had built up a relationship with the researchers and might therefore have felt that they could be more honest in giving their scores on the second occasion. This is pure speculation but seems plausible. As always, methodology is a key issue in interpreting the results of a piece of research.

Training needs to be pitched at a level that takes into account the existing knowledge and experience of the carers. Information packs and medical input are highly valued and carers identified a need for more in-depth specific training. In another project, Professor Klein reported that the need for information about ADRD was repeatedly identified in the carer literature of many EU countries [29].

The H.O.M.E. project concluded that social support **is** an important factor in the health and well being of carers. Notice that although it is clearly judged as significant, the amounts of social support actually reported by carers was unrelated to their stress levels in our own sample of carers in England. However, we assessed social support with questions such as "Do you have people around you who help you to keep up your courage?" and "Do you have at least one friend or relative whom you can really trust?" The H.O.M.E. study, on the other hand, included practical help like respite care, day care and home care as a part of social support, and so it mixed services and social support together. Once again differences in methods and definitions probably help to explain these different findings.

The H.O.M.E. study identified other forms of support that are valuable in helping carers maintain their caring role more effectively and for longer and at less personal cost to themselves. Examples are:

◆   Acknowledging the difficult task of caring

◆   Countering isolation

◆   Emotional support

◆   Learning through information and training

◆   Helping with finding and using sources of support

The H.O.M.E. study also pointed to the need for:

◆   Larger scale evaluation of the impact of education and

training on quality of life for both carers and people with dementia.

- The development of thinking and communication skills in hearing the voice of the person with dementia.
- Improving support for informal carers.
- Early diagnosis so that effective interventions can be made as early as possible.

Professor Klein's study complements the findings of the H.O.M.E. study. A training package was devised to deal with the forms of support that the H.O.M.E. project identified. The training package was designed for leaders of support groups and for families of people with ADRD and is available in 11 EU languages and on CD. The training package is composed of seven modules:

1 **General Recommendations for Group Leaders**: how to design and run a carers' group.

2 **Information:** dementia; legal and financial matters and ageing.

3 **Support**: use of services, social support; the group as a mutual support system.

4 **Cognitive Emotional and Behavioural Changes of Person with Dementia**: dealing with memory loss, changes in communication and concentration, dealing with anxiety/fear, depression or apathy, dealing with aggressive or agitated behaviour, sleep disturbances, hallucinations and delusions, inappropriate sexual behaviour, wandering and restlessness, inappropriate incontinence.

5 **Increased Dependency of Persons with Dementia**:

home care skills, activities of daily life, safety issues, falls, incontinence.

6   **Impact of Disease on Carer**: anxiety, loneliness and isolation, guilt, positive aspects of care.

7   **Self Care**: stress management, relaxation, taking time for oneself, leisure/free time (for care and person with dementia), making plans for the future.

Another project organised by the Training, Teaching and Support Group[5] provided a general framework for designing training programmes and methods for evaluating them. One example is a Spanish programme which aims to respond to the feelings, emotions, wishes and needs of the person with dementia. There are eight sessions in which family members learn to:

♦   discover the needs and wishes of the person they are caring for and their own needs and wishes.

♦   recognise and analyses the possibilities and restrictions of the older person, themselves and their surroundings.

♦   respond to the needs and wishes of the person with dementia and to create conditions for the development of new-life activities and social relationships within the possibilities.

A Swedish programme, 'Living with Dementia', by Associate Professor Gertrud Grahn and Professor Barbro Beck-Friis, is an educational programme for formal as well as informal carers[26]. It is based on what carers, and especially informal carers, have suggested are important knowledge and skills for the creation of optimal conditions regarding the patient's functioning and well-being, and to be able to assure dignity for the patient, handicapped by dementia. The evaluation of the course has been published in Swedish (Grahn, 1998).

Carer manuals

In order to help carers to deal with dementia various books and care manuals have been written. The recent manual by Alzheimer Europe[9] enables the carer to find out how to deal with the changing needs of a person with dementia and discusses how to cope with caring. An example of advice given by Alzheimer Europe is given in Box 5.5:

Box 5.5:   How to cope with eating and drinking

Provide assistance if required, without taking over unnecessarily or causing embarrassment.

Encourage independence.

Give the impaired person plenty of time and try to make mealtimes a pleasant experience.

Try not to worry too much about correct manners and tidiness.

Adapt the mealtime situation to the needs of the impaired person (the routine, the utensils, the kind of food served, etc).

Ensure that he/she drinks 1 and a half litres (8 cups) of water per day (to avoid dehydration and increased confusion).

If he or she seems to have lost his/her appetite, contact a doctor to determine whether there is a physical cause and whether nutritional supplements are needed.

Consult a dentist to determine whether dentures, gums or teeth are causing pain and hence interfering with eating.

Source: Alzheimer Europe's Self-Help Carer Manual[9]

Madame Flori and her team studied care needs in Germany, France, Italy, Portugal, the UK and Sweden[17]. It was found that the elderly population was broadly researched, mostly during the 1980s, with scientific and popular publications focusing on patient treatment and care. However it was found that in these countries there is little or scattered availability of official information on the needs of elderly persons suffering from dementia. The perception of needs is often intuitive, with no systematic search for information. Furthermore, surveys are often not representative[17]. Further systematic research is needed in order to have a better understanding of both the carers' needs and the needs of the people they are caring for. Studies carried out over time (longitudinally) will enable a better understanding of the changes that occur in patterns of care as the disease progresses and the family learns to deal with dementia.

Gaps and resources in health care systems in the European Union

Professor Klein and his collaborators[29] found that the resources available to carers differ considerably across the EU. The gaps identified by Professor Klein and his team came from reports made by national co-ordinators following literature searches. Their findings offer some insight into the gaps in ADRD care in the EU.

In general, it was found that, with some extensions, there is a decline from the north to the south in caring for carers. The highest standards were found in the Scandinavian Countries and the Netherlands. The situation for families was found to be worst in Greece and Portugal. On the other hand many specific problems were reported from most European countries especially from Belgium and Ireland where there is a great need for improved services.

Denmark reported a lack of geriatric specialists and a lack of support and interest from GPs. This holds true for many other countries that also criticised the role of the GPs. In the Scandinavian countries the resources from the health care system are very good but this does not mean that there are no problems. A lack of social support is frequently reported in the northern countries whereas in the southern countries more support and respect for elderly people were found but less respite care.

Some countries, for example Italy, reported strong regional differences in the quality of health care within the country. Especially in rural areas carers lack qualified personnel and institutions. Researchers in Greece stated that there is no real interest for people with ADRD. In rural parts of Greece the deficits in ADRD care are very severe. In Spain and other southern countries there is an under-usage of self-help groups.

In Austria, despite the fact that GPs are the first contact person or gatekeeper for the carer and the person with dementia, they do not give adequate information. In Belgium there are only a small number of care facilities available. In Finland informal carers receive a monthly allowance of 3-400 Euro. These payments provide at least some token recognition of the tasks that informal carers perform.

Societies and cultures vary according to the degree to which they value the interests of the individual as a self-contained unit versus the interests of the family, group or community. These two forms of society are referred to in cultural anthropology and sociology as "individualist" and "collectivist" respectively. In reality, no society is entirely individualist or collectivist; all societies contain a mixture of both tendencies.

In countries and regions in the south (e.g. Portugal, Spain, Greece, and Southern Italy) where they believe strongly in the role of the family and the community, they paradoxically do very little to assist families who are dealing with dementia. This may be because dementia still remains largely unrecognised as a disease and is wrongly seen as an inevitable feature of ageing. Once again there is a strong case for more public education to modernise these perceptions.

Conclusions

The current picture for informal carers across Europe is rather grim. Although there are oases of excellent provision and good practice, the overall scene is patchy and inadequate. There are no common policies, agreed principles, or minimal standards. What happens when a person is diagnosed with dementia is dependent on local and chance factors. In most of Europe the resources to support carers and sufferers appear to be inadequate. The principal carers are predominantly female, unpaid, and unsupported, an 'invisible' labour force motivated by love or loyalty. Carers with a strong sense of coherence cope better with their stress than others. The findings from the Middlesex/EACH and EUROCARE studies suggested that neither formal support nor social support is correlated with the informal carers' stress levels. This could be for one of two reasons. Either these two support sources are normally too slight, or they are not targeted sensitively enough, or there could be a mixture of the two. Further studies using a longitudinal methodology with larger, representative samples are urgently needed. On a policy level, more collective responsibility needs to be taken at community and societal levels if millions of informal carers are to enjoy a higher quality of life.

KEY TERMS

Carer burden

Carer stress

Cross-sectional survey

Informal care

Prospective design

Sense of coherence (SOC)

CHAPTER 6:   FORMAL CARE

"Recognise the person having dementia as a subject living in relation to others. Find ways to be, to live with and to care for this person."

Source: A Training programme for the carers of people with dementia by the Training, Teaching and Support Group[5]

Usually a person with dementia comes into contact with a range of professionals and volunteers during the course of the illness. This type of care is known as "formal care". The amount of contact with formal carers varies according to the needs and wishes of both the person with ADRD and the informal carer. It will also depend very much on the local circumstances and conditions. Examples of the professionals who are likely to be encountered are doctors, nurses, care assistants, gerontologists, social workers, psychologists, psychiatrists and dieticians. In addition many organisations that support carers rely on the services of volunteers.

Although the basic aims are similar, the relationship between people with dementia and the professionals, volunteers and informal carers who provide care for them is different[5]. For professional carers, their occupational role and the organisational framework in which they work define the relationship with people with dementia. This can mean that contradictions or conflicts sometimes arise in the relationship between a professional carer and a person with ADRD. For volunteers, the relationship with the person with ADRD is based on voluntary choice and so it is freer from professional or organisation rules and principles. Therefore the role of the volunteer is a more independent one. Both the person with

ADRD and the volunteer can end the relationship whenever they want to. For an informal carer a relationship already existed before ADRD. They care for all different kinds of reasons: out of love, because they want to, feel an obligation to do so, because they think that 'everyone' expects it from them, or simply because there is no one else.

An important idea is the **continuum of care**. This means that the care someone receives in one setting should carry over into another. A wide range of people must meet the needs of the person with dementia. Communication is not an easy task between so many different people and may lead to a breakdown in the continuum, differences of opinion and sometimes even to conflicts. For example, a doctor and a dietician may decide that a person needs to increase their iron intake owing to drug therapy having caused slight bleeding in the stomach. However the care assistant who helps the person at mealtimes knows that she does not like liver, kidney, red meat, or nuts. Therefore rather than find alternative sources of iron, the care assistant allows the person to continue eating cakes as she wants to allow the person with dementia to choose her food.

In order to ensure that there is a continuum of care, it is important that professional carers communicate with one another and, if possible, meet on a regular basis. Also informal carers need to be fully included as involving professional carers in the care of a relative or friend can sometimes make informal carers feel excluded, out of control or guilty (Marshall, 1996).

Care Settings
Formal care takes place in a variety of settings, e.g. in a residential home, in a day care centre, in a specialised care unit,

or in a hospital. Quite often different philosophies exist in these settings. However it is possible to discern some general 'design principles' for good practice in dementia care, as we shall see. The ETAS project[30] defined ten different arrangements for care. In addition to these, expert centres and specialised care units (SCUs) must be added. A list of settings/arrangements for dementia care is shown overleaf in Table 6.1.

Table 6.1:   Settings and Arrangements for Dementia Care

Settings	Arrangements
Home care service	Domestic support, domiciliary nursing, auxiliary nursing
Primary care teams	General practitioner, nurse therapist, assessment and care planning
Social care	Social workers, assessment and care planning
Day care	Support worker in own home, social care, hospital-based
Respite care	In own home, unit/centre
Secondary service	Psychogeriatrician, geriatrician, neurologist, psychologist
Expert centre	Multidisciplinary team for assessment, care planning and follow-up
Specialised care unit	Residential units specialising in dementia care
Nursing homes	For-profit, charitable

Hospitals	Psychiatric units, geriatric and general
Residential homes	State (decreasing), for-profit, voluntary, religious
Voluntary sector	Domiciliary, support workers in own home

The Salmon Group[25] is a network of organisations throughout Europe that provides small housing units for older people as alternatives to large institutions. It aims to provide support according to the needs and choices of older people responding in a flexible and practical way to individual differences. It therefore takes into account culture, disability and mental health. The Salmon Group[25] has analysed ways in which small housing units can be adapted in every respect to offer flexible and personal care in the community to dementia sufferers. The Salmon Group believe that similar principles can be applied to caring for people with dementia and caring for older people in general. However they also point out that including people with dementia in such residences can cause tensions. One such tension is between family and staff who would like to minimise the risks to people with dementia and the Salmon Group's belief that residents should be allowed to take risks.

Specialised care units (SCUs) have been developed in several countries to improve the care of patients with dementia. In 1994 the regional government of Lombardy in northern Italy set up a comprehensive system called "Piano Alzheimer" which aimed to take care of patients in different phases of AD (Bianchetti et al, 1997). Of particular interest was the possible reduction in severe behavioural problems. Dr Giovanni Frisoni of the Gruppo di Ricerca Geriatrica in Brescia, Italy conducted a case control study of the efficacy of special care units in France and Italy in the improvement of quality of life of patients and their relatives[19]. In Dr Frisoni's evaluation, specialised long term care and acute care was compared to conventional long-term and acute care. It was found that specialised units enhanced the quality of life of patients by reducing behavioural disturbances without resorting to pharmacological or physical restraints. The improvement in behavioural disturbances was not significantly different from that achieved in traditional wards but the amount of physical restraints prescribed and used was found to be much lower. The benefits on behaviour persist over time and were observed for at least three months after the initial evaluation. Changes in falls, cognition and disability were not clinically significant in either specialised units or traditional, control wards. This study suggests that specialised institutional care can help reduce the use of costly pharmacological interventions (Frisoni et al, 1998). This brings us to an important topic: the concept of person-centred care.

Person-centred care

Person-centred care takes into consideration that people with dementia are individuals with their own unique needs. It allows for the fact that before a person develops a dementia they have their own unique experiences and personality. The late Tom Kitwood was a leading worker on person centred care for people with dementia. He said that:

Instead of seeing a set of deficits, damaging and problem behaviours awaiting systematic assessment and management which effectively turn the person into an object, we need to work on the basis of seeing the person as a whole. This does not deny the presence of a dementing illness but sees it within a context that is social rather than medical[27].

According to Kitwood (1993), in adopting a person-centred care approach for people with dementia, barriers between "we" and "they" are dropped. As well as discovering about the person with dementia, we can also discover ourselves. It makes us realise our common humanity.

Goldsmith (1996) points out that when people develop dementia, it is always in the context of a unique personality and that it is necessary to understand as much as possible about the person you are relating to when caring for someone with dementia. Goldsmith highlights the fact that dementia is an umbrella term for a range of different conditions and that each one has its own specific pattern and characteristics. People with Alzheimer's disease have different needs from people with vascular dementia or Creutzfeldt-Jakob disease or disabled people with dementia[26]. Culture, race and class add to these differences so that, for example, people from ethnic minorities have different needs from those in the ethnic majority[15].

Goldsmith (1996) states that:
Lumping people together under the label of 'dementia' and approaching them in the same way is likely to increase the problems of communication and make it more difficult for us to hear their voices.

The person-centred approach to care is all about trying to hear the voice of the person with dementia. If someone never liked watching television and always preferred to read a book, they are likely to become quite frustrated, angry and uncooperative if a carer puts them in front of the television. Rather than accept the frustration and anger as part of the dementia, it is necessary to look further and try to identify what is causing the frustration and anger. This can be quite time consuming and challenging for the carer and a lot of effort can be required. However it can make caring easier in the long run and more satisfying (Goldsmith, 1996).

A key part of using the person-centred approach is to learn about the person's life history, tastes and preferences. Faith Gibson (1993) has discussed the use of the past in working with dementia patients in the present: "Our sense of identity, self-esteem and personal confidence is largely rooted in our knowledge of where we have come from to whom we belong" (p. 40). Gibson believes that our sense of wellbeing stems in part from our knowledge of our past and that this is also important for people with dementia whose memories are more ambiguous, hazy, and intermittent. She suggests that a detailed knowledge of the person's past becomes the means by which "we extend our capacity to venture, to explore, to remain a travelling companion for more of the journey and postpone for a time the parting of ways" (p. 43). Reminiscence is an effective way of building a life history and thereby understanding the person as a unique individual (see Chapter 7).

Faith Gibson (1993) recommends the use of reminiscence techniques and observations as a means of painting a picture about the life history of the individual in which the "rich colour and texture of a person's life could be sketched". Fine-grained detail of the person's life can be gathered, e.g.:

◆ Did the person like to have their hair permed?

- Did they like a soft or a hard pillow?
- Did they use an alarm clock?
- Were they interested in clothes?
- Did they like jewellery?
- Did they eat sliced or unsliced bread?
- What were their hobbies and interests?
- Were they houseproud?
- Who was their favourite film star?
- Where had they lived/worked/holidayed?
- Who had been their significant others?
- Who was still likely to be significant?

The recognition of the person with dementia is a key principle of the person-centered approach and fundamental to good practice.

Good Practice

What is good practice? New approaches to services for people with dementia are continuously developing throughout Europe. Professor Mary Marshall and her team at the Dementia Services Development Centre, University of Stirling, Scotland, in association with E.A.C.H.[04, 11] collected data on care providers' views on good practice. The Stirling/EACH team also investigated the extent to which respondents felt their services were able to comply with these views on good practice. It was concluded that no service is entirely good but every service has some good points. Some of examples of 'design principles' for good practice in dementia care can be seen in Box 6.1. Full details of these design principles are available from the Dementia Services Development Centre's WebPages (see Box 7.2, Chapter 7).

Box 6.1: **Principles of Good Practice in Dementia Care**

These four principles are selected from a larger set suggested by Mary Marshall:

Small: A small scale is helpful to people with dementia and their carers. People with dementia have impaired learning and reasoning skills so a reduced amount of stimulation and information is clearly what is required. A small scale is also likely to promote greater knowledge of the individual and their carers, which is also likely to be helpful. Unfortunately cost constraints may force providers to care for people in larger groups, e.g. residential homes.

Properly designed: The design should:
◆ compensate for disability
◆ maximise independence
◆ enhance self esteem and confidence
◆ demonstrate care for staff
◆ be orientating and understandable
◆ reinforce personal identity
◆ welcome relatives and the local community
◆ allow control of stimuli.

The features of good design are:
◆ small
◆ familiar
◆ domestic
◆ homely in style
◆ with plenty of scope for ordinary activities
◆ unobtrusive concern for safety

- different rooms for different functions
- age appropriate furniture and fittings
- safe outside space
- single rooms big enough for lots of personal belongings
- use of clear signs
- use of objects rather than colour for orientation
- enhanced visual access
- control of stimuli
- especially noise

Trained, supported and respected staff and volunteers: Staff and volunteers need to be trained constantly in knowledge, skills and attitudes. They do a very difficult job and need the tools to do it well.

Given the emotionally and physically demanding nature of the work, it is also important that staff and volunteers feel well supported by their management.

Based on the knowledge of the individual: Without a knowledge of the individual, good care is impossible since people with dementia are often unable to easily communicate their needs and wants or even to say who they are.

Source: European Alzheimer Clearing House - Good Practice. Workpackage 2. Workpackage Leader: Professor Mary Marshall (4)(11)

Optimal living at home

The European Dementia in Family (EDIF) project[31] aimed to stimulate support for family carers in their efforts to create an optimal living situation at home. The study examined how patients and their families can deal adequately with problems of dementia at home and how specialist services for geriatric patients can be integrated into community services. The study was conducted at three sites in Spain, Belgium and the Netherlands. All participants agreed on a standard set of inclusion criteria for the target group, methods and instruments.

At a time when institutional care is being replaced in many national policies by care in the community, there is growing interest in "transmural" care. Transmural care is a term used for providing professional care in community settings rather than in hospital. Transmural care follows these basic principles:

◆ Provision of major help (informal and formal) in a community setting before the decision of out-of-home placement is made

◆ Offering tailored services to the needs of the patient and the primary carer (family-centred planning)

◆ Combining various in- and out-patient services and various skills, training and knowledge of staff about dementia in one team

◆ Providing specialist services in constructive interaction and communication with home help services and the general practitioner

The study by Meindert Haveman and René Reijnders [31] was designed to evaluate the extent to which it is possible for a transmural team to:

◆ Mediate and ameliorate the objective and subjective "burden" of care for primary informal carers

◆ Prevent (progression of) physical or psychosocial consequences to carers

◆ Let patients stay longer with their informal carer and provide other residential choices (e.g. day care, respite care, senior homes) than nursing home placement by offering extra support and services within a comprehensive programme

◆ Delay the progress of dementia symptoms and problems with social skills and roles compared to those receiving the usual services provided in that region

The study design was a randomised field study design. In each region a minimum of 50 patients were randomised into two groups resulting in 25 patients for the transmural intervention group and 25 patients in the control group. Overall this meant that 75 patients and their informal carers participated in the intervention and 75 in the control group. Baseline measurements were taken and then outcome measurements 3 and 6 months after randomisation.

Social psychogeriatric services and GPs recruited patients in the three regions. Patients with Alzheimer's disease, vascular dementia, or other types of dementia with scores of 5 or 6 on Reisberg's GDS scale (see Chapter 1) were eligible for the project. Persons on a list for nursing home placement within three months or in the terminal stage of dementia were excluded. The average age of the participants was 76 and one third of the sample was male, two thirds, female.

Baseline measurements on the person with dementia consisted of the Cambridge Examination for Mental Disorders in the Elderly (CAMDEX) (Roth et al., 1986), the Activities of Daily Living (ADL) scale, the Instrumental Activity of Daily Living Scale (IADL) and the Rapid Disability Rating Scale-2 (RDRS-2) (Linn & Linn, 1982).

Baseline measurements on the carers consisted of the Sense of Coherence Scale of Antonovsky (1987) (see Box 2 for more details), a measure of objective 'burden' from the Time Demand Scale (Heller & Factor, 1991) which assesses the total amount of time the carer is spending on helping the person with dementia from 0 to 60 hours a week, and feelings of depression on the Hamilton Depression Scale (Hamilton, 1960).

The results of the EDIF project showed that the randomisation turned out to be quite successful; the distribution of almost all of the prognostic variables being equal between the intervention and the control group. The final numbers in the intervention and control groups were 57 and 59 respectively. The average age for the central carers was 62 years for both groups. Half were partners, and the other half were children or other relatives. The principal carers were spending 5 to 8 hours a day directly on caring tasks in relation to the person with dementia and 1 to 3 hours on household tasks. The results suggested that the transmural programme, which had provided social support and care to the principal carers, did not have a significant effect on the SOC or Hamilton Depression Scale individually. However, the generalised effect of the two variables together did appear to show a significant effect of the intervention. A further analysis suggested that the positive outcome of the intervention had a stronger effect on younger carers aged 26 to 54 than on older carers aged 71 to 84. This was a well-controlled study with excellent matching of participants between the treatment and control groups. It is unfortunate that the number of cases could not have been larger so that more definitive results could be obtained. However these results are encouraging and suggest that transmural support can have a positive outcome on the wellbeing of the principal carers.

Raising the status of dementia care through improvements in training

Mary Marshall (1996) points out that despite the fact that dementia care is an exciting and developing field that is open to new ideas, it is still a low status field to work in. Many people working in dementia care are unqualified and there is a lot of poor practice. The hard work that people working with dementia do often goes unrecognised. Despite the fact that dementia is on the increase and often takes a member of a family out of the workforce, it is also still not yet a health service or policy priority.

These issues have been addressed by some of the Alzheimer's projects reviewed here, especially conference projects that often invite political figures to participate. This is a good way of helping politicians and policy makers to understand the complex array of issues that concern people working with dementia[1,2,11,21,23]. Another way of enhancing the status of dementia care is to improve the training of health professionals.

A group of researchers from Belgium have worked on a project called "Te Deum: A transcultural educational dementia project for Europe."[12] The Te Deum project recognises that early as well as the correct diagnosis of dementia is an essential element in successful care provision. People with dementia and their relatives are becoming an important element in the workload for general practitioners. Therefore, GP's knowledge about dementia is very important.

The Te Deum researchers reviewed studies that give a differing picture to the existing knowledge general practitioners have about dementia. For example one study by Bowers in 1992 found that primary care physicians in country areas had more restricted knowledge and limited insight into the causes of dementia. In an interview study 50% scored poorly on a knowledge test. However an Australian study published by Henry Brodaty (1994) showed that GPs had a reasonable knowledge of the clinical picture of dementia and the problems of the carers.

Several reasons are put forward to explain different findings about doctors' knowledge. As previously mentioned, different studies use different methods for collecting their information. This makes comparisons difficult. Some studies use postal questionnaires, others use personal interviews while some use indirect methods like the patient's judgement. Also the state of GPs' knowledge clearly varies from country to country.

The Te Deum researchers designed an interactive computer based training programme for doctors to learn more about dementia. The programme consists of five modules, each modules is presented as a case study. Active participation is required through a simulated patient case. The user has to answer questions in each module. The progress of users is registered and access to the next module is only possible if all chapters of the previous module have been explored.

The Te Deum project evaluated the effort needed to adapt the training programme to the specific linguistic, cultural and health care background of different European countries. The development of a structured educational programme of electronic courseware is itself very labour intensive, time consuming and costly. Collaboration between educationalists, experts, information technology advisors and/or software engineers is needed. An important point was also raised by this project. Simple linguistic translation of the content of the programme is not enough to make it suitable for the professional communities in other European countries. Knowledge of the culture, the society and health care system of the country is needed in order to translate effectively. Any national expert group can use the Te Deum programme as an initial blueprint but the involvement of different national expert groups is required at every further step of the development process.

Other projects have used the more traditional method of seminar training for professionals. Jacques Selmes and his team from EACH [11] designed a training programme for professionals and volunteers to educate informal carers about Alzheimer's Disease. The project aims to be transcultural and suitable for use in each European Union member state. Versions in English, French and Spanish have already been published. It is flexible, as it is adapted to the different levels of knowledge of the trainers. The essential notions of an educational programme called "The Educational Programme for Alzheimer's principal caregivers (EPAC)" are presented to the potential trainers along with "selected reading" for each theme. This allows trainers, in combination with their own experience and familiarity with the theme, to deepen their knowledge. There are 34 overheads necessary for the presentation of the EPAC programme as well as short case studies. They are also given information on structuring training seminars for future group leaders. This is all directed towards the aim of having a wide diffusion of this training tool.

The issue of nursing care is very important for people with dementia and their families. Adequate staff training is a basic necessity for improving the quality of life of people with dementia and their carers. Presently in the European Union levels of nurse education vary across countries which makes it not only difficult to compare the qualifications of the nurses in different countries, but also restricts mobility. Given the European Union's, attempt to guarantee freedom of movement of labour, this is an important issue. It is an issue that the Dutch members of E.A.C.H. [11] have addressed.

Professor van Londen and Ans Grotendorst obtained details on the level of qualifications of nurses in different EU member states (Belgium, Denmark, France, Germany, The Netherlands, Spain, Sweden and the UK). They recommended approaches to improve the comparison of qualifications and the impact of training programmes on dementia care. They point out that even when a lot of money and time is spent on education and training of professional carers, the results can often fall short of expectations. The carers learn a lot on the course but the new knowledge and skills are not applied in the work environment. Box 6.2 lists recommendations of EACH concerning these issues.

Box 6.2:   **Recommendations for Enhancing the Impact of Training Programmes on Dementia Care**

---

1   A systematic approach
Health care organisations and trainers should meet each other before training takes place to answer the following questions:

◆   Which results do we want to achieve in our organisations?

◆   How must the work environment function in order to achieve those results?

◆   Which skills do managers and nurses need to create such an environment and realise good dementia care?

- Which learning situations do we need to design?
- Do the learning situations enable trainees to achieve the desired learning results?
- How can we test the trainees' proficiency?
- Have the trainees applied their new skills in the work environment?
- Is the work environment receptive to the new skills?

2 Creating a shared vision among stakeholders

The process must be clearly understood by all that play a role in making it successful: managers, experienced nurses, teachers, etc. A useful technique is creating a diagram that highlights the critical roles, interactions and results needed to achieve performance improvement. This technique focuses the attention on the total system, rather than each separate programme. Everyone can see how training interventions become transformed into positive results for dementia care.

3 Comparability instead of uniformity

Uniform assessment criteria and comparable degree requirements are still needed but it is to be recommended that more attention should be paid to diversity in health care services and educational systems. Rather than putting the focus on quantitative elements and vainly trying to equalise structures and systems, it is desirable to move towards diploma comparison based on competencies.

Source: European Alzheimer Clearing House - Nursing qualifications in different EU member states. Workpackage 7. Workpackage Leader: Prof.drs J van Londen

As well as improving their knowledge about dementia, it is just as important for formal carers to adopt a person-centred approach (see Chapter Five). This was one of the objectives of The H.O.M.E. Project - Helping Older people with dementia be Maintained at home through Education and training[27]. This project developed a training programme for formal carers in Northern Ireland that was underpinned by the person-centred approach to care (Kitwood 1993).

When this training programme was evaluated, several interesting issues were raised. The H.O.M.E. team[27] believed that the programme would have been better if the training had been done jointly with informal carers to facilitate learning between groups and to enable information exchange. Future work should also be done in obtaining user views about service provision (see Goldsmith, 1996). The home care workers positively evaluated the training programme. The H.O.M.E. team[27] stress that this kind of training should not be seen as an event, but every effort should be made to encourage home care workers to see this as an ongoing developmental process. In other words, the training is not just a day event that allows absence from work, but a form of professional development that enables better work to be done in future.

The reality of formal carers providing a person-centred approach to care may not be so simple. After the intensive 8 day training (that included courses on communication skills, person-centred care, role of caring and workers' expectations, understanding behaviour) home care workers in the H.O.M.E project[27] were placed with people who had dementia living in their own homes. The home care workers found that their time and resources were stretched to meet the needs and practice of a person centred approach to care. They were often visiting one client 7 or 8 times each day. This was not practical as they could be quite a distance away and the worker did not always have transport. This can be very exhausting for the formal carer. Despite this the H.O.M.E. team felt that the home care workers' participation at this early stage was vital. Their views on the service were regularly fed back to management via the training so that resources could be created and maintained. Fortunately the manager of this service was able to respond to these viewpoints and action was taken.

This brings us back to the beginning, resources for people with dementia are not a political priority. Our own survey findings suggested that the current services and resources available to informal carers in England are not significantly related to the stress levels of the carers either because they are too slight or because they are not being well targeted. While there can be little doubt that the majority of people working with dementia are doing their very best with limited resources. They often are felt to provide a "lifeline" by many carers of people with dementia. Services should be need led rather than demand led.

Further research is needed to confirm that a person-centred approach to care is beneficial, not only to the person with dementia and to the carer, but to society at large. Then the political will needs to be found to allocate resources to implement these research findings.

Conclusions

Finding good ways of organising dementia services is becoming an increasingly active area. Of key importance is the person centred approach, treating the dementia sufferer as a person first and as a dementia sufferer second. Another key principle is to aim at a continuum of care, a reliable and stable regime of care across all settings and providers, whether informal, professional or volunteer. Dementia services development centres are a valuable resource of information and expertise to all those engaged in seeking and providing good practice. Transmural care is provided by expert outpatient centres that can liaise with all relevant parties in providing support to families and dementia sufferers. Much later in the progression of the disease, specialised care units are able to deliver high quality care that maximises freedom and minimises the use of drugs and/or physical restraint.

KEY TERMS

Continuum of care

Dementia services development centres

Person centred approach

Specialised care unit (SCU)

Transmural care

CHAPTER 7: COMMUNICATION AND INFORMATION

Les échanges se réduisent au fil du temps et la communication est de plus en plus difficile à établir. Alors que faire? S'armer de courage, apprendre à connaître la maladie pour accepter d'appartenir à des mondes différents et garder la force de rechercher et encourager tout ce qui peut encore être partagé malgré tout: quelques mots, un regard, un sourire, une caresse...

Translation: Exchanges become less frequent as time goes by and communication is more and more difficult to establish. So what can be done? Arm yourself with courage, learn to be familiar with the disease in order to accept belonging to different worlds and keep up spirits to find out and encourage everything that can still be shared despite everything: a few words, a look, a smile, a caress...

Soucre: Quoted from 'Daily life info' April 1997

The issue of communication and information in the field of ADRD covers several areas. Firstly, professional communication and the care of people with ADRD will be explored. Secondly, communication in relation to the person with ADRD will be discussed. Thirdly, public domain sources of information on dementia will be described.

Communication between professionals

As already mentioned in Chapter Six, many professionals are involved in the care of a person with dementia and it is essential that communication between them is effective if there is to be a continuum of care. Often, the professionals involved in care come from different disciplines. This has many advantages to offer. Care becomes more holistic, as the person with dementia is viewed from different perspectives. However professionals need to be careful when they are working in multi-disciplinary teams. Different professions have different languages, and so, when they initially work together, confusion and conflicts are not uncommon. It is very important for multi-disciplinary teams to try to establish a common language and common goals. Otherwise a well-thought out and well-intentioned care plan can often go wrong due to poor communication between professionals.

In order that a person-centred approach to care prevails, good records need to be kept, updated and read by professionals. Records should ideally be made on conversations and advice given to family members and friends in order to prevent mixed messages. It can be quite upsetting for people close to the person with ADRD to receive advice from one professional that totally contradicts the advice from another. It can make them feel confused and worried and can cause conflicts in the care team. Records should also include as much history as possible so that a picture of the person can be built. Records might include information on past employment details, family, likes and dislikes, religion and cultural background. A system of good record keeping is not always in place. However Mary Marshall (1996) states that in the UK, records are improving all the time.

It is crucial for professionals working with people with dementia and their carers to have good communication skills. Sometimes communication is the only route to information about someone's physical and/or mental state. Effective communication can sometimes be therapeutic in itself (Marks, Murray, Willig & Evans, 2000).

However communication between a health care professional and a lay person can also be a complicated process. Let's take the example of a carer going to see a doctor about the person they are caring for. The doctor may use words that seem quite natural to her but the carer might not understand and be reluctant to ask for clarification or may be so lost that they do not know how to ask for a better explanation.

The carer probably has her or his own ideas and beliefs about the problems associated with dementia that may well differ from the doctor's. These ideas may be related to culture, religion, reading of newspapers and magazines, or experiences from everyday life. For example, one carer might not be willing to fully accept that their relative has dementia because their relative has always exercised, had a healthy diet, never used an aluminium pan (even though this is probably not a risk factor) and always been rather religious. The carer believes that all diseases are related to unhealthy diets and lifestyles. The doctor, on the other hand, believes that the relative has dementia because she is 85 and has obtained a low-score on the mini-mental. The carer may then leave the doctor feeling dissatisfied, unable to retain any information that the doctor has given, and perhaps even untrusting. The carer will think twice about going to see the doctor again. Yet from the doctor's perspective, she/he is simply 'doing their job', oblivious of any problems.

It is therefore vitally important that health care professionals learn how to use language that is clear. This requires health professionals to be aware of lay theories of health and illness and to be able to translate their own medical explanations into everyday language. Mitchell and Cormack (1998) present some ideas for good communication for practitioners that apply equally well to professionals working with people with dementia (see Box 7.1).

Box 7.1:   Good Communication

1 Good communication should aim to take place in the context of a respectful and caring therapeutic relationship. The health care professional should:

   ◆ negotiate an authentic relationship which may change over time and which is suited to the needs of the particular individual.

   ◆ listen carefully to what is being communicated (with words and body).

   ◆ offer support, encouragement and realistic hope.

   ◆ be sensitive to emotional states and needs.

2 The health professional should try to find out about beliefs about health and illness. This can be done by clarifying views about:

   ◆ what might have caused the illness/incident?

   ◆ what the future might hold?

   ◆ what might be needed?

3 The health care professional should try to explain their point of view, at a pace and level which is relevant. They should explain their views about:

   ◆ the cause of the problem.

◆ what is recommended.

◆ what self-help activities can be undertaken.

◆ expected outcome of treatments/interventions

4 Good communication includes trying to understand the person's experience of the consequences of their problem. Attention should be given to accounts of the history of problems.

◆ what are the important events and relationships in his/her life?

◆ what consequences does the problem have for his/her life?

5 Clear, open and respectful communication provides a framework for shared understanding which will change and develop over time. This may enable the person receiving advice to:

◆ decide whether the advice is relevant for his/her needs.

◆ make use of the advice because it has been explained in a way which is relevant to his understanding.

◆ feel helped by the health care professional's support, understanding and acceptance.

Source: Mitchell and Cormack, 1998

Communication and the person with dementia
Breakdown of language is one of the symptoms of Alzheimer's Disease. Many people believe that communication with people with Alzheimer's disease is a huge problem or completely impossible. However this view is

changing and people such as Malcolm Goldsmith (1996) believe that communication with people with Alzheimer's Disease is possible and should be encouraged.

The EUROCARE study [34] found that loss of language and communication were the aspects of dementia that spouses found the most difficult to cope with. This is supported by a review by one of the authors (Marks, 1998) that found that the inability to hold a sensible conversation was one of the aspects of dementia which carers found most difficult to deal with. Problems with communication can cause carers a great deal of frustration and often lead them to ignore the person the dementia.

Interventions have been designed to deal with communication problems. Goldsmith (1996) states that certain 'basic ingredients' need to be in place before enriching the process of communication. The person without dementia must be able to listen and accept the person as they are and accept the possibilities of communication.

Music has been used to help communication with people with dementia. Gôtel and Ekman presented the results of one such programme at the Alzheimer's Disease International Conference[23] in 1997. It was found that when people with dementia were taken to the toilet while music was playing they showed more ability and seemed to be more alert than without music and actually said that they like listening to music during toilet time. The carers also communicated more, both verbally and non-verbally, with music than without music. When singing together people with dementia seemed to be even more alert and communicated more than when listening to music.

The Alzheimer's Disease International Conference[23] in 1997 included several presentations about communication. Saarela Merja from the Finnish Association on Mental Retardation presented research on games as an aid for interaction in dementia care. It was found that the introduction of games in a residential care home changed the behaviour of people with dementia. They became less anxious and aggressive. There was increased concentration on activities and increases in shared interaction among people with dementia. The staff learned more about the strengths that residents still possessed. However there appeared to be difficulties with shared interaction between residents and staff. Although the amount of interaction increased, the interaction was lacking such qualities as intense attention, shared joy and equality. This finding highlights what Goldsmith (1996) says about the 'basic ingredients' needed before attempting to improve communication.

Reminiscence work

Reminiscence work is another type of therapy that can improve communication with people with dementia. Age Exchange [32] in London organised a conference for the European Reminiscence Network in which different aspects of reminiscence were discussed. Faith Gibson (1998) described reminiscence work as seeking "to help the person retain a sense of who they are and to remain in relationship with others by identifying common ground and creating shared identities." Reminiscence is about using imagination and sensitivity "to find ways of communicating which enrich, confirm and encourage people to remain in relationship with others and in this way remain in touch with themselves." Reminiscence work focuses upon the long-term memory, as this part of the memory remains comparatively intact in most forms of dementia. Faith Gibson points out that various means can be used in reminiscence such as music, drama, dance and movement, painting, story telling, writing and reading. When reminiscence is guided with a trained listener, it becomes therapy (Forster, 1998).

Reminiscence work can take place in a variety of settings for example hospitals, nursing and residential homes, social centres, day care centres and people's homes. It can be done with individuals or small groups. However many people with dementia do better in one to one relationships. Effective reminiscence groups need to be small. Triggers such as pictures, artefacts, sounds, tastes, smells, events, trips, music and animals can all produce a great deal of interest and shared conversation. In order for reminiscence work to flourish in formal care settings, there must be an ethos in place which values people as individuals, creates opportunities for them to live in community with each other, and perceives dementia care as attending to the whole person and not just to their physical care and safety (Gibson, 1998).

Bob Woods also spoke at the conference for 'The European Reminiscence Network' and focused on reminiscence and communication. He argued that dementia care workers who carry out reminiscence work communicate powerful messages to the people with dementia. Here are a few examples of these messages:

We value you as a person.

The whole person's life is of interest in reminiscence work, physical care is not the only priority. Reminiscence work reminds carers that they are caring for a living person, with a lifetime of experiences and emotions.

We are interested in you as an individual.

Carers take a genuine personal, non-judgemental interest in the person with dementia and their life during reminiscence.

We respect you and your experience.

In reminiscence work each person's life is respected and considered to be rich and varied.

You know things we can never know.

During reminiscence the carer asks questions to which s/he does not have all the answers, and which will be forever outside his/her experience. It is the person with dementia who is the expert.

When we know you better, the gaps in our understanding become less.

A person's attempts to communicate may not always be understood by the carer. However once the person with dementia is known as a whole person the more fragments become clear and complete.

I am an individual

In reminiscence work the person's individuality gradually breaks through.

My life story is part and parcel of who I am now.

A person cannot be understood in isolation from all that she has experienced. A person brings to dementia her preferred ways of coping with difficulties, which may have a large impact on how she behaves in the new situations that she now encounters.

Bernie Arigho gave examples of reminiscence work at the European Reminiscence Network conference. He described the Age Exchange Reminiscence Project that took place at White Gables Day Care Centre in Bromley. One such example firstly involved the participants using a ball and name game. A ball is thrown and the person who catches it has to say their name. This game helps to break ice and involves everybody straight away. Then a tray of reminiscence objects was passed around the group and the participants were invited to choose an object. They were asked to contribute some information about what the object was, including memories that it brought back for them. The session ended by reviewing and appreciating in a positive manner everyone's contributions. The participants were asked what they would like to do next week. Arigho points out that although this may produce many practical ideas, it sets the right tone of respecting the guests and giving them power and control within the group.

Bridget Penhale and her team at the University of Hull, UK, have produced a template of good practice in reminiscence groups[24]. A summary of these guidelines is presented below:

♦ When starting a reminiscence group it is important to remember that preparations can be time consuming and need a lot of effort.

♦ Many different types of permission may be required from trade unions, politicians, higher administrators, employment offices and the county labour board. In the Swedish model of a welfare state there is very little experience of voluntary work and it is therefore more complicated to start a reminiscence group with volunteers.

♦ It may be difficult to find volunteers for a reminiscence project. You should be prepared to look for new solutions. Volunteers need a comprehensive training, not only about dementia, reminiscence work and group processes but also in communication skills.

♦ You have to decide what subjects should be discussed and what triggers should be used. Old photographs are a good trigger. A stressful atmosphere can be created if you know that you have to work through a certain number of subjects and triggers. There must be possibilities for changing themes spontaneously.

♦ Not anyone has the necessary skills and experience to start a reminiscence group. To run the group you need management skills and ability to deal with difficult situations. You need a lot of negotiation skills and administrative skills to be able to get all the different types of permission and support you need. You also need good knowledge about reminiscence work, dementia, knowledge about helpful literature in these fields in order to train and supervise the group.

♦ Supervision of the volunteers should ideally be done at least after every second session.

♦ It is important to get a good start to each session.

♦ It may be a good idea to start with a drink. This creates recognition and a sense of community, which helps all the members of the group to relax.

♦ The composition of the group is of great importance. Sometimes it is better to work individually with some of the participants, some people may have tendencies to dominate the group. This confirms the theories that not all people are suitable for reminiscence groups. Staff need to have knowledge for each participant when structuring the groups. People who dislike each other have a tendency to dominate each other or irritate each other. They should not be put in the same group. It is also useful to have some participants whose memories are more intact. Such individuals can stimulate the other participants in a way that younger volunteers or staff cannot do by talking about old times and common memories. Another thing to remember when starting a group is that there are great differences between the participants when it comes to which part of life they remember. Some of them can only remember their childhood, some have a clear limit later in life, while others only remember separate fragments from different times. it is important to reflect over this when structuring the group. To ask a key worker to join the group can provide great support and security for a participant but it can also have the effect of holding the participant back.

♦ The spatial arrangements are of great importance. Sitting around a big table makes it difficult to hear what is said at the other end of the table and difficult to see the triggers. Subgroups develop.

♦ Make sure the sessions are not too long. Even if some of the participants do not want to leave the session, the majority becomes tired and inattentive after about an hour.

♦ Ensure sustainability. It is not ethical to start a reminiscence group if sustainability cannot be guaranteed if the work is successful.

◆ Evaluation should be done when all sessions are completed. To sit down and in a relaxed atmosphere and discuss what has been good and what went wrong is a very good practice in order to make the next group function even better. Evaluation is a way to improve the knowledge in the field both for the supervisors of the group as well as for all involved and also for the theoretical development of the field.

Information about dementia in the public domain

When a family member or friend is diagnosed as having dementia, it is usual to want to know as much as possible about dementia. Professor Klein's project found that carers usually want information about the disease, financial support, caring services and organised emotional support[29]. All Member States have an Alzheimer's Association where information and advice can be obtained (see Part 3 for details). All these associations are members of Alzheimer Europe[2, 3, 9, 10].

Alzheimer Europe is a European-wide organisation that aims to:

◆ promote by co-operation the support of patients suffering from Alzheimer's Disease, or related disorders, and their carers.

◆ raise awareness of Alzheimer's Disease by the medical profession, paramedical organisations, social services and the European Commission and European Parliament.

◆ exchange information between the national Alzheimer societies.

◆ develop models for improved care of Alzheimer patients.

◆ increase political advocacy in each of the member countries and centrally with the European Commission and Parliament.

◆ promote the training of personnel caring for Alzheimer patients.

◆ encourage and support research and the advance of knowledge into the cause, early diagnosis, treatment and prevention of Alzheimer's Disease.

◆ promote world-wide co-operation with other organisations having the same or similar objectives and in particular Alzheimer's Disease International.

Using an Alzheimer telephone helpline is one way of obtaining information and help. Alzheimer Europe (AE) has written a telephone helpline manual that offers advice on setting up helplines[3]. An Alzheimer telephone helpline should be accessible to everyone (e.g. carers, professionals, media, people with dementia); confidential; ideally accessible 24 hours a day; providing immediate help or advice at a low cost to the caller. The main aim of an Alzheimer helpline is to provide a person to talk to, who knows the difficulties due to personal or professional experience.

For people with access to the Internet, there are lots of useful web pages about Alzheimer's Disease. Many of these sites have links to others. A few examples are given overleaf in Box 7.2.

Box 7.2:   **Dementia web sites on the Internet**

Alzheimer Europe, Luxembourg:
http://www.alzheimer-europe.org

Alzheimer's Disease and the European Union:
http://www.alzheimer-europe.org/eu.html

**Dementia Services Development Centre
University of Stirling, Scotland, UK:**
http://www.stir.ac.uk/dsdc

Dementia Web:
http://dementia.ion.ucl.ac.uk

**European Alzheimer Clearing House
Brussels, Belgium:** http://www.each.be

**Health Education Research Unit
University of Cologne, Germany:**
http://www.uni-koeln.de/ew-fak/
For-ges/Alzheimer/alzheimer.html

**Middlesex University Health Research Centre
London, UK:**
http://www.mdx.ac.uk/www/jhp/ecad.htm

**The Special Care Unit for People with Dementia
Italy:** http://www.unibs.it/~grg/scud/index.html

Université de Rennes, France:
http://www.MED.UNIV-RENNES1.FR

Conclusions

It can be seen that effective communication together with a desire to understand is a vital element of dealing with dementia. The provision of multiprofessional dementia care requires making special efforts of communication as does communicating with people with dementia. As much energy as is put into promoting treatments and interventions needs to be put into improving communications skills. Without these basic skills, treatments and interventions cannot be expected to reach their maximum potential. Some basic ingredients need to be in place before the process of communication can be enriched. The person without dementia must be able to listen and accept the person with dementia as they are and accept that communication is a possibility. Communication involves listening, hearing and observing as much as speaking. Reminiscence work stimulated by music, drama, dance and movement, painting, story telling, writing and reading and playing games promotes the enjoyment of shared social interactions and the retention of a personal identity that is both meaningful and purposeful. Alzheimer's associations provide valuable resources through information, advice, support groups, conferences, helplines, web sites, training of volunteers, and political advocacy.

KEY TERMS

Alzheimer Europe

Alzheimer Disease International

European Reminiscence Network

Reminiscence work

CHAPTER 8: TREATMENTS AND INTERVENTIONS

Although there is no medical cure for dementia, the situation for the dementia patient can be improved using treatments and interventions. In this chapter we describe and discuss the options that are currently available in the light of recent evaluations. These options fall into two broad categories: (i) Drug treatments that (a) slow the progression of the disease; (b) treat conditions associated with dementia, e.g. depression; (ii) Non-drug interventions. It is generally agreed that a multidisciplinary approach to the management of dementia is the most likely to provide best for the patient's needs.

In the next section, we will present a brief description of how the theory behind the drugs' action and briefly describe each of the available drugs. The research that has been conducted on the drug effects on the symptoms of AD will not be covered here as it is beyond the scope of this book. However we summarise the main effects of each drug including side effects. Following that we review the efforts that have been made to develop non-pharmaceutical interventions.

Drug treatments

The cholinergic hypothesis

The cholinergic hypothesis assumes that acetylcholine (ACh) metabolism plays a role in memory processes of storage and or consolidation. It is assumed in this hypothesis that degeneration of cerebral presynaptic cholinergic neurons causes deterioration of memory and other cognitive functions. The theory is based on the evidence that choline acetyltransferase (CAT) is deficient in autopsy material from AD patients. From the so-called "cholinergic hypothesis" four kinds of drugs have been tried:

◆ ACh precursors: Patients have been fed large doses of choline or lecithin in an attempt to compensate for the reduction of internally generated choline. In spite of a lot of hype in the media in the 1980s, this strategy has failed to produce any reliable, positive results.

◆ ACh releasers: Patients have been given drugs that will promote the release of ACh such as aminopyridine and 3-4 diaminopyridine. Some limited success has been obtained.

◆ Direct acting ACh agonists: Drugs that act on either the muscarinic or nicotinic receptors of ACh have been administered e.g. xanomeline or galanthamine. The latter is an alkaloid found in the bulbs of snowdrops and several other plants of the genus Galanthus. These drugs are showing promise and are being hailed as the "next generation" of AD therapeutics. However we must await the outcome of properly controlled randomised trials before we get too excited about this possibility.

◆ Choline-esterase inhibitors: This approach has been a major strategy in the 1980s and 90s and has led to a large amount of research. We discuss the application of these drugs in the next section.

Acetylcholine-esterase (AChE) inhibitors

When the pre-synaptic terminals of cholinergic neurones release acetylcholine, AChE removes a large part of the acetylcholine (ACh) from the synapse so that its effects are only short-lived. In AD it appears that a large number of cholinergic neurones are destroyed so that the amount of acetylcholine that can be produced is also decreased. Thus by reducing or inhibiting the AChE should make it possible for ACh to remain longer in the synapses and allow better transmission of neuronal impulses. This theory has led to the approval of several AChE inhibitors (AChEIs) manufactured by pharmaceutical companies. This is in fact the only class of drugs with any clinically proven efficacy in AD patients. All drugs need to go through a number of stages of evaluation before they can be registered and approved for use. There are two major registration agencies, the Food and Drug Administration (FDA) in the USA and the European Medical Agency Administration (EMEA) in Europe. Drugs have two names: a generic name and a brand name. The generic name is the official medical name for the basic substance (e.g. donepezil) and the brand name (e.g. Aricept) is chosen by the company that produces the drug.

The profile of an ideal AChEI is as follows:

◆ Provides a meaningful clinical benefit
◆ Is well tolerated
◆ Is highly selective
◆ Has no organ toxicity
◆ Has no adverse cardiovascular effects
◆ Has minimal drug-drug interactions
◆ Does not induce or exacerbate negative moods
◆ Does not impair memory
◆ Has a simple, flexible dosage

The basic idea behind the use of AChE inhibitors is to delay the progression of the disease compared to the situation that would occur without use of the medication. This is illustrated in Figure 8.1. The decline in mental function that occurs without treatment is shown in the lower curve. The delay in this decline that can be brought about by taking a drug that inhibits AChE is shown in the higher curve. It can be seen that a delay of six months or even longer can in principle be achieved in this way. This in turn could delay the need for the person with dementia to leave the family home and move into an institution.

Figure 8.1:   Delaying the intellectual decline in AD using an AChE inhibitor

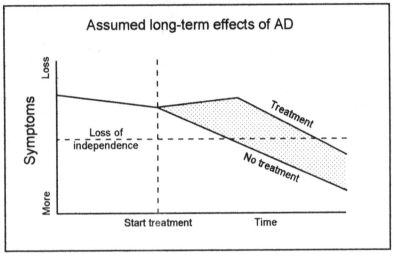

Source: Adapted from Feldman & Gracon, 1996

Three drugs are currently on the market, but more drugs are likely to follow. Each new drug appears to be an advance on the previous ones. Perhaps the day will eventually come when progression of AD can not only be temporarily delayed but also stopped completely. That will be a breakthrough worthy of the Nobel prize because we will finally have a cure for dementia. Until then, this small group of AChE inhibitors are the only drugs that can be recommended specifically for the treatment of AD patients.

Tacrine or COGNEX

Tacrine is a chemical substance with a very long name: 1-2-3-4-tetrahydroaminoacridine (THA). This drug was the first to be registered and to reach the market. It was approved initially in the USA and France and subsequently in 25 other countries including the UK, Sweden and Denmark. However the drug was not marketed in all countries where it had been approved, e.g. in the UK. The drug is given four times a day and the dosage is gradually increased from 10mg every six weeks. The optimal dosage of 160 mg/day can be reached after about 5 months, although not all patients can tolerate this dosage and the maximum tolerable level varies from person to person.

Adverse side effects include nausea, vomiting, diarrhoea, increased sweating and bradycardia. Its use must be avoided in patients with known liver disease. There is the possibility that there will be changes in liver function which, fortunately, can be reversed when the dosage is ceased. This results in dramatic increases in liver enzymes of up to 10 or 20 times the normal limits. The toxicity to liver function is a major disadvantage as is the need to administer the drug four times a day. It also shows a tendency to interact adversely with other medications.

Donepezil or ARICEPT

This drug was specifically developed for the treatment of AD. It was the first drug marketed for AD in the UK. It has low liver toxicity while generating a similar effect on the core symptoms of AD. The much improved safety/efficacy profile of donepezil suggested that an advance had been made in therapy of AD. Two main doses are used, 5 or 10 mg. The most common side effects are gastrointestinal (nausea, diarrhoea and constipation) but these are mild in intensity and transient, lasting only a few days. However there have also been reports of skin rashes (Bryant, Ouldred & Jackson, 1998). The effect on cognitive function is also fairly minimal, the highest dose tested (10 mg) showing less effect than that reported for the highest dose of tacrine.

The drug was the subject of controversy and debate in the *British Medical Journal* (BMJ) in 1997. An advertisement for donepezil (Aricept) breached the advertising code and did not give a balanced view of the data, the Prescription Medicines Code of Practice Authority ruled. The advertisement published in the BMJ and other medical journals was headed "Mum has Alzheimer's" beneath which appeared a large coloured photograph of an elderly woman and her daughter, both smiling. Beneath the photograph, running on from the heading, it said, "but she knew I was calling today". An appeal board decided that the advertisement gave the false impression that the patient's memory had improved after treatment with donepezil. Stein, Milne and Best (1998) reported on a review that they conducted which concluded that donepezil is a "borderline case" yielding small benefits at relatively high cost. Boothby et al (1998) argued for a national policy or guidelines for prescribing the drug because there has been such varied practice across different parts of Britain. In some places it can be obtained on prescription while in others it is deemed too costly.

Jones, Mann and Saunders (1998) contacted 62 chemist shops in and around the English city of Bath to find the cost of a one-month prescription of donepezil, 5 mg and 10 mg. The NHS cost in 1998 was £68.32 for 5 mg and £95.76 for 10 mg. The costs charged for a private prescription (paid for by the patient) varied from £68.32 to £120.41 (average £98.66) for 5 mg and £95.76 to £168.78 (average £139.18) for 10 mg. In general they found that local chemists that were not part of a chain quoted the lower prices. The authors discovered that the higher figures were nearer to Pharmaceutical Society guidelines that suggest that the retail price should include a 50% mark up on the actual drug price plus a dispensing fee. Jones, Mann and Saunders comment: "These guidelines seem more applicable to the pricing of wine by top restaurants than to the health needs of patients with dementia, and such profiteering is surely unacceptable." They suggest that patients and carers should be warned by their doctors to choose their pharmacist with care and check the price beforehand.

Rivastigmine or EXELON®

This is a new AChE inhibitor that is selective for the target enzyme, AChE, in the cortex and hippocampus, the brain areas most affected in AD. It has a chemical name that is usually abbreviated to ENA 713 (rivastigmine tartrate) and the brand name is Exelon®, a registered product of Novartis Pharmaceuticals. Rivastigmine mimics ACh as a substrate for the enzyme AChE which stops further destruction of ACh in the synapse. This means that neural transmission is made easier and the symptoms of AD can be successfully reduced. The effect of one dosage lasts for approximately ten hours.

The efficacy and safety of the new Alzheimer drug have been demonstrated in an international study (ADENA) with 3,300 patients. Two dose ranges of 1-4 mg per day and 6-12 mg per day were compared over 26 weeks to a **placebo** in a **randomised double-blind design**. The efficacy of treatment was evaluated on three criteria: cognitive function, global rating, and activities of daily living (ADL). Standard methods for measuring these three indicators of treatment efficacy were used. The results showed that patients showed a small but significant improvement in cognitive function over the 26 weeks on the high dosage of Exelon® while those on the placebo showed a significant decrement. The clinical effects of the drug were reported as early as 12 weeks after administration.

As a part of the ADENA study, Corey-Bloom et al (1998) conducted a randomised trial of ENA 713 on 699 patients with mild to moderately severe probable AD. 235 patients were assigned to a placebo group, 233 to a low dose of 1-4 mg per day, and 231 to a higher dose of 6-12 mg per day for 26 weeks. The AD patients receiving the drug were found to show a lower decline in cognitive function than the placebo group. In several trials reported in the manufacturer's Product Monograph including the one reported by Corey-Bloom, safety and tolerability appear to be good. People in the trials were elderly with no upper age limit (average age, 72 years), had concurrent illnesses (in more than 85% of cases) including cardiovascular problems, were receiving other medications (73% of people) and were mostly living at home. The most common side effects were nausea and vomiting but, according to company reports, these effects were transient and mild-to-moderate in intensity occurring at initiation or when the dose was increased. There also appeared to be very low risk of interactions between Exelon® and other medications.

Evidence is needed from open field trials on the extent of the delay in AD progression that can be obtained with this and other AChEI drugs. The results from the large-scale clinical studies are encouraging and we look forward to further developments.

Non-drug interventions

Drug treatment is only one part of the totality of ways for dealing with dementia. Effective methods for managing the disease need to consider both the patient and their families. There are also "psychosocial interventions" in the form of therapy and counselling that are designed to improve the functioning and quality of life of people with dementia and their carers. These consist of

◆ Memory training programmes

◆ Use of memory aids

◆ Reality orientation

These techniques attempt to compensate for the cognitive decline. Psychiatric and behavioural complications of ADRD also occur in 90% of patients and these include:

◆ Depression

◆ Delusions

◆ Wandering

◆ Aggression

These symptoms can also respond well to behavioural and environmental interventions, in addition to any therapy provided in drug form. Among the EC funded projects, two were concerned with reminiscence work and described in the previous chapter. Another was concerned with interventions to support memory. We describe this project in the next section.

Individualised memory aids

Dr Fred Furniss at the University of Leicester has been collaborating with COO.S.S Marche, a social services group in Ancona, Italy to run a pilot scheme on developing individualised memory aids for people with AD[28]. The aim of the project was to develop simple memory aids, tailored to the individual, in order to prompt appropriate language. These were to be used in the every day living environment of the dementia sufferer. This work was based on the earlier findings of Bourgeois (1990, 1992, 1993) who showed that the use of simple memory aids enhances the quality of conversation of people with moderate AD. These memory aids consisted of photos, pictures and simple descriptive sentences depicting areas where the patient had been experiencing memory difficulties. As would be expected, the effects were strongest with less severely impaired AD sufferers.

The Leicester/COO.S.S group repeated the intervention used by Bougeois with five people with moderate to severe dementia (Mini-Mental State Examination scores 0-12). The project evaluated the impact of the memory aids on the proportion of the time spent in conversation that the participants could remain on the topic. Furniss found that seven participants increased the proportion of conversation that they spent on the topic when using the memory aid by up to 100%.

In one part of the project (Study 1) the team observed day to day influences on the speech of five people with dementia in a nursing home. Each person was observed during three 90-minute sessions during late morning in a lounge/dining room of their residential home. The behaviour of the person with dementia and other relevant persons was recorded using a Psion hand-held computer. It was found that physical proximity of staff or visitors was important so that when another person was within 5 feet of them, people with dementia were five times more likely to engage in conversation than when they were alone or with another resident. The study led to three conclusions:

(i)   it is helpful to organise patterns of staff working to maximise the time staff spent in physical proximity to residents.

(ii) approaches to encouraging conversation between residents should be considered.

(iii) the patterns of staff-resident interaction during activities of daily living warrant further investigation to determine which kinds of interactions are associated with higher amounts of conversation.

Study 2 evaluated the quality of conversation of persons AD when talking about topics which carers had suggested would stimulate conversation. The same five people participated but this time in the afternoons. Each participant was engaged in three sessions of conversation by a carer for periods ranging 7-20 minutes. The carer directed the conversation to at least two different topics, one classed as "personal", which the staff believed the participant liked to talk about, and another as "control", which had been identified as one which the participant was not generally interested in talking about. The results were very variable depending on the person and topic. There appeared to be no consistent differences between personal and control topics, which seems a little surprising.

Study 3 examined the conversation of five persons with dementia living in family homes as well as in protected homes. The study designed a questionnaire for the formal and informal carers to identify issues that might stimulate conversation. A meeting was held with the patient's family and formal carers. An observation of one hour of interaction between a carer and the patient was carried out and recorded. The content of the interaction was classified as: on-topic, out of topic, unintelligible, incorrect, ambiguous sentences. The elements of conversation were also classified according to the domain:

- Affective: issues relating to people who have, or had, an emotional impact on the patient

- Objects: all tangible elements, e.g. dresses, pictures

- Remembrances: places, events, music and songs of the past, i.e. situations stimulating remembrances such as place of birth, where they lived in their youth

- Dynamic-physiological: confusion, food, pains, age

- Other: elements that could not be classified under the above

The study attempted to identify the possible memory aids for each patient and to provide general guidelines on how to build up the aids and how to use them.

The elements of the conversations fell mainly within the Affective (5 patients out of 5), Remembrance (3 out of 5), Objects (2 out of 5), and Others categories. The role of the family in stimulating the participants' conversations was very evident. It was concluded that it would be best to focus possible aids on photographic material consisting of relatives and pictures or postcards showing places of birth/youth. Furthermore the presence of carers is a major stimulus to conversation in people with severe dementia.

Guidelines for developing and using memory aids
Memory aids are aimed at improving the conversational skills of people with dementia. A memory aid should be

made individually for each person. Typically the aid consists of a memory wallet consisting of photographs, pictures and simple sentences. However the aid could be a poster, a box, a stand-up presentation card, or any other form of presenting personal information, e.g. an audio tape for a person who has a visual impairment. The following aspects need to be considered[28]:

♦ Emphasise positive memories

♦ Be aware of memories that the person may not like to talk about

♦ Select simple, important events and information

♦ Choose things that will promote conversations and communication

♦ Make the aid as clear as possible but visually appealing

♦ Make a copy of any photo/article prior to use

♦ Designate a certain place where the aid should be kept when not in use

Items to include in a memory aid include:

♦ Photos of family, friends, pets, etc

♦ Postcards from favourite places or holidays

♦ Small items from a hobby, e.g. stamps, parts of a train set, a medal

♦ Pictures of famous people

♦ Short newspaper articles, clippings, etc

♦ Favourite ornaments

♦ A tape of a favourite piece of music

All of these stimuli and objects are the kind of memorabilia that anybody would keep for sentimental or nostalgic reasons, so there is nothing particularly special about these procedures. It takes some special care to construct a memory aid for another human being instead of doing it for oneself. Furniss and his colleagues found that all participants with severe dementia consistently produced substantially more on-topic conversation when using memory aids than in phases without the aids. Not all participants produced a dramatic change initially, and so their aids were reviewed and modified to provide greater memory support.

Conclusions

Drugs that improve neural conduction in the cholinergic system of the brain are able to delay the progression of AD. However these drugs are expensive and they also have side effects. For these reasons they are not being prescribed by all doctors everywhere and so, once again, we see evidence of inequalities in treatment across regions and countries.

There is a need for implementation of policies within Member States to ensure more equal treatment opportunities for dementia patients within and across nations in Europe.

KEY TERMS

AChE inhibitor (or AChEI)

Aricept (donepezil)

Cognex (tacrine)

Design

Double-blind

Exelon® (rivastigmine)

Memory aids

Multidisciplinary approach

Placebo

Psychosocial interventions

Randomised

CHAPTER 9: POLICY AND EQUITY

According to Kitwood (1993) 'much is loaded against' the rich possibilities of person-centred care. He pointed out that: "The 'epidemic of dementia' is occurring while society is in a deep economic crisis, and when the social structure that might sustain good caring are not in place." We will now be looking at policy issues that help provide the social structure to better deal with dementia. Issues concerning equity and economics of dementia care will also be discussed.

We saw in Chapters 5 and 6 that there are no common policies, agreed principles, or minimal standards of care across Europe. There is little equity in dementia policy for European citizens. What happens when a person is diagnosed with dementia is dependent on local or chance factors. In most of Europe the resources to support carers and sufferers are inadequate or inaccessible. The provision of good services to support carers is therefore a matter of some concern. Better services for informal carers can be justified on economic and social grounds as well as an ethical concern with fairness and equity.

It was suggested by the EUROCARE project[34] that less than half of the carers interviewed were receiving any formal assistance raising questions "about the accessibility of formal services and indeed in some countries about the need to develop appropriate forms of domiciliary care and respite provision" (p. 25). Other issues raised by this study were the low numbers of families in contact with support groups and associations, the stresses that appear to result from financial dissatisfaction, the need for flexible employment conditions, tax incentives, advice and information, and the overall need to create a more positive public image of dementia.

In spite of a general feeling that dementia care has had a "Cinderella" status and that something significant must be done at a policy level, there is also a feeling that only lip service is being paid to the issue (Johansson, 1998)[16]. In part, the lack of activity by national governments is justified on the grounds that dementia care is one component of "care in the community" that occurs at the level of counties and municipalities. Another reason for inactivity of national governments has been the divide that exists in many countries between health and social services, with dementia care running between the two umbrellas and getting a rather poor deal from each system. It is helpful to consider policy and practice relevant to informal care for people with dementia in two countries, Sweden and the UK.

National Policies in Sweden and the UK
The information in this section is drawn from reports at a French seminar on Alzheimer's disease at INSERM, Paris, in December 1998 by Dr Lennarth Johansson (Stockholm, Sweden) and Professor Sally Furnish (Manchester, UK)[16].

Sweden: Swedish national policy is to guarantee older people a secure economy, adequate housing, social services and health care according to their needs. Laws and regulations mandate local governments to provide services and care to their citizens. Health care is the responsibility of 289 municipalities and social care the responsibility of 23 county councils. These services are predominantly financed by taxes and the user only has to pay a fraction of the total cost. Local governments levy their own taxes and decide how they wish to spend their resources independently of national government.

Sweden has been experiencing a swing away from an emphasis on formal care provided by the state towards informal care in the family. Service contraction has occurred since the 1980s and there has been an increasing gap between resources and needs. In 1988 a government proposal focused on the goal of replacing institutional care with less costly alternatives. This was the first time in Swedish elderly care policy that special attention had been given to the need to support informal carers. "Care leave" was implemented in 1989 giving family carers the right to a paid leave from work of up to 60 days to care for a family member especially in cases of terminal and acute care. In 1992 this concept was extended to allowing care leave to be reimbursed from social insurance when visiting a person who is ill in hospital.

In 1990 the Ädel reform transferred responsibility for care of the elderly to the municipalities, providing considerable advantages of co-ordination, and placing the responsibility for supporting informal carers in the hands of the municipalities. In 1997 the government provided extra funding for projects aiming to develop new models for supporting informal carers. This extra support appeared to be necessary following research on the high stress levels of carers in which carers in Sweden were found to experiencing heavy demands and receiving little or no support.

Three kinds of support are currently available in Sweden:

◆ Economic support: carers can receive attendance allowance paid to the dependent to pay the family member for her help. This is a "modest" sum of at most SEK 5,000 per month. Persons under 65 (of "working age") can also receive a carer's allowance in which the municipality reimburses the carer for her work. Finally, there is payment of care leave for terminal situations only.

- ◆ Respite care: in 1997 there were 6,282 beds available for institutional respite care in Sweden (4.6% of all institutional beds). There is also the possibility of adult day care, there being about 600 units in Sweden in 1995.

- ◆ Counselling and personal support: support groups usually run by voluntary organisations are now available in the majority of municipalities. Some limited amount of counselling also is available.

In addition to the use of adult day care centres, people caring for Alzheimer's and other dementia sufferers, 60 or more dementia nurses or dementia teams carry out outreach activities to support families. A few experimental schemes are employing home-helpers and voluntary organisations also provide special services to support carers such as sitting services, support and training groups and helplines.

Experience with the above systems of support suggests that there has been only mixed success. In 1996 care-leave was used by about 6,500 persons, only half of those who were eligible, and these were principally employed women around age 50 looking after people with terminal cancer. The economic recession has restrained the impact of the Ädel reform on support to carers. Almost none of a random sample of 70 municipalities had an explicit policy for supporting carers although almost every municipality could offer respite care and economic support programmes. It seems clear that the general policy of municipalities is to offer services rather than economic support to family carers. The numbers receiving economic support have been declining over recent years.

In spite of the care of the elderly being one of the hottest publicly debated issues in Sweden, Dr Johansson concludes that it has been more a case of "lip-service" than actions. Perhaps new legislation debated in the Swedish Parliament in the Autumn of 1998 may lead to more effective carer support and a balance will be found in "optimising family and public resources, in a partnership in care" (Johansson, 1998)[16].

United Kingdom: The conservative government's NHS and Community Care Act 1990, implemented in April 1993, identified specific outcomes, established a new framework for services, and developed an agenda for management and efficient use of resources. As in Sweden, local authorities were given the lead role in social care. The outcomes of community care under the Act included:

- Enabling people to live as normal a life as possible in their own homes or in a homely environment in the community

- Focusing provision on those in greatest need

- Tailoring packages of care to the assessed needs of individuals

- Maximising the independence of individuals

- Restricting interventions to the minimum to achieve independence

- Giving service users a greater voice

- Providing practical support for carers

Eligibility for local authority funded social care was means tested. Individuals could retain savings up to a maximum of £16,000. A charge for domiciliary and/or day care may be levied to eligible individuals. The maximum cost to the authority is usually the equivalent of the cost to the authority if the individual entered residential care. Social services must target resources at those with greatest need and so this means targeting those who live alone or for health or frailty reasons are at greatest risk. Social care funding therefore tends to be spent on personal care (washing, dressing, etc) which are considered essential if elderly people are living alone and want to stay in their own homes.

The new labour government's agenda to modernise health and social care has four themes:

◆ It links with the wider agenda to deal with social exclusion by tackling the root causes of ill health, including social and economic factors. Whether carers will be included in the drive to reduce social exclusion remains to be seen but it could be argued that there is a very good case.

◆ Breaking down the barriers between services through partnership working across agencies.

◆ Ensuring uniformly high standards and maximising value for money.

◆ Making services faster and more convenient.

Funding mechanisms for continuing care for people with dementia in the UK await the outcome of the Royal Commission on Long-term Care.

Professor Furnish[16] concludes her review with the statement that "Despite ample evidence of the effectiveness of interventions for carers, the future direction of policies for carers in the UK is unclear." While families are not under any statutory duty to provide care for an elderly relative, they often feel a duty to provide direct care, putting at risk the family savings. Furnish states: "Keeping the person with dementia in contact with their carers, without exploring those carers, should be an underlying service aim. Services are not innovative enough to be fully responsive to that aim."

Principles of national policy

The policies of the European Member States relating to dementia have been reviewed in two EC projects: The Transnational Analysis of the Socio-economic Impact of Alzheimer's Disease in the European Union[33] and the European Transnational Alzheimer's Study (ETAS)[30]. These two studies produced a considerable amount of information and we summarise here their main conclusions and recommendations very briefly.

The ETAS report summarised the key principles that underlie public policy. These policies appear to have been driven by both politico-economic and humanitarian concerns. Key principles that have emerged in all Member States are:

♦   People with dementia should be enabled to remain at home for as long as possible.

♦   Carers should receive as much help as possible in order to facilitate the above.

♦   People with dementia should retain maximum control over the support they receive.

♦   All relevant services should be co-ordinated at the local level.

♦   People with dementia in institutional care should live in surroundings which are as 'homely' as possible.

Principles that have been emphasised by most Member States are:

- There should be a systematic attempt to equate service provision with need.

- Categorical care should be replaced by care that addresses the general needs of sufferers.

- Early diagnosis of dementia should be encouraged.

- The needs of people with dementia are addressed only as part of the approach to older people in general at the national level.

The ETAS report suggests that the 1990s were a period of consolidation during which criticism has focused only the policy framework and on the perceived inadequacies of its implementation. According to the report, criticisms of implementation (or its lack) of national policy have emerged in most Member States because of:

- Continuing lack of adequate resources, particularly resources 'ear-marked' specifically for this client group.

- The persistent relatively low status of dementia services in the broader context of healthcare.

- Inadequate attempts to ensure patient and carer control of services, which remain largely shaped by organisational and professional imperatives.

- The health and social needs of patients and carers still do not always receive equal attention.

Legislation

The ETAS report states that none of the Member States has enacted legislation relating to the specific needs and circumstances of people with dementia. People with dementia and their carers are governed by more general legislation. Legislation is discussed under two headings: that relating to individual rights of people with dementia; that relating to the overall control of services.

Individual rights

Where matters of property require resolution. Some states (e.g. The Netherlands, UK, Ireland) have provision for enduring powers of attorney, or 'living wills'. These allow people to determine in advance how they wish their property is to be administered, and by whom, before they cease to be able to control it adequately themselves. Other states (e.g. Finland, France) do not have this provision, and seek means of administering the property of people with dementia in a way that might best have met their wishes after dementia has progressed.

When giving consent to treatment. General mental health and other legislation is applied by most states when necessary to compel people with dementia to receive treatment, under appropriate safeguards. Until the point when individual choice and responsibility is removed, many states have legislation to enforce the patient's right to choose between different forms of treatment. In some states however (e.g. Luxembourg) specific legal guarantees of individual autonomy for people with dementia are apparently absent.

When seeking access to medical and other records. Many states have moved to provide certain rights of access to one's own (and a demented relative's) medical and other information.

Provision of services

The ETAS report classifies legislation under this heading into three broad forms:

Permissive   agencies are empowered to act to meet certain needs, but the manner and extent to which they do so is left to their discretion

Prescriptive   certain types of provision are required

Regulatory   where certain types of services are provided and the standards of that service are regulated by law

The ETAS study found that most states have a mixture of all three with wide variations between countries. The Netherlands has high standards of institutional residential care that are enforced by law. Some states (e.g. Finland, UK) have statutory provision for patients' complaints procedures.

Policy recommendations

The two transnational studies made a series of recommendations concerning improvements in policy and practice. Many of these echo and reinforce the conclusions already reached elsewhere in this book.

The LSE report[33] recommended more dissemination of information at European, national and local levels concerning: assessment of carer needs, the importance of advocacy in service delivery; increased awareness of dementia and dementia services; improved education and training of professionals; social protection of carers; stimulation of debate; and promotion of the importance of carers.

The ETAS report[30] identified a number of key issues and recommendations relevant to the EU as a whole. Of particular importance were the following issues:

◆   **Dementia sufferers and their carers are treated**

inequitably among Member States

Among other things the ETAS report recommended that: there should be a concerted effort to use the most effective means of public education to change negative attitudes towards dementia, and in particular to emphasise the benefits of early diagnosis. The professional status of healthcare staff working with people with dementia should be increased.

◆ **There is inequity within and between Member States in dealing with dementia**

The report recommended that the European Commission should work with the Member States to provide assistance to those countries where dementia services are furthest from the ideal level. The Member States should improve the consistency of local application of recognised good practice.

◆ **Intervention often occurs at too late a stage in the progress of dementia**

The report recommended that the relevant agencies in each Member State should:

(i) develop an effective strategy to increase the level and quality of assessment and diagnosis of ADRD at the early stages of the disease; (ii) ensure that general medical and allied professional education included sufficient input on dementia at undergraduate, postgraduate and continuing education levels.

◆ **ADRD policy should be co-ordinated and services multidisciplinary**

Member States should continue to address the need to improve co-ordination – at the policy and implementation levels- to meet the total needs of AD patients and their carers.

◆ **Carers of dementia sufferers require better support**
There should be further improvements in the systematic identification of the needs of carers, supported by the allocation of adequate resources to meet their (often-modest) requirements. All Member States should continue to improve the mechanisms used to involve carers in the planning of services.

(In listing the above points we have amended the authors' original references specifically to "Alzheimer's disease" or "AD" to the more inclusive and generic terms of "dementia" or "ADRD").

Equity

So far we have seen that equity issues need to be addressed for people with dementia and their carers. Dementia does not receive as much recognition as other major diseases. But imagine you are a 50 year old Algerian man living in rural Greece and you start to experience the first signs of Alzheimer's Disease or a 30 year old woman with learning difficulties living in Sweden and dementia creeps up on you. You would experience even further inequity. Inequities of care and quality of life exist among people with dementia. At present, if young people, residents of rural areas, ethnic minorities and people with learning difficulties in the European Union face dementia, they also face even further inequity.

Some projects have been undertaken to start to tackle these issues. The ENIDA project also has done work in the field of people with learning difficulties and dementia. [13] A video and brochure in French and Dutch were produced. Issues covered include: How do formal and informal carers perceive dementia in older people with learning difficulties? What are the signs and symptoms to look for? What types of care and support are appropriate for older people with learning difficulties who develop this disease? The relationship between Alzheimer's Disease and Down's syndrome and useful caring techniques were also covered. The video is warm and shows a person-centred approach. It provides a great deal of information and allows the spectator identification with the various situations shown. The brochure is pocket-sized and the language is clear. The ENDIA project drew up a dissemination strategy and the video has been shown at various seminars in France, the UK and Holland. An article about the video appeared in the medical newspaper Quotidien du Médecin.

'The world of dementia is colour blind and minority communities are dementia blind.' This statement by Professor Mary Marshall sums up the situation for ethic minorities with dementia. Dementia does not discriminate between races. Yet there is an inadequacy of provision of care and recognition of dementia amongst ethnic minorities. The Stirling/EACH[11] project conducted a survey of the situation of service provision for ethnic minorities with dementia. Replies such as 'Minorities? We just had not thought of them...but now that you mention it we think it is relevant...' or 'We don't have any minorities...' were not uncommon replies from service providers in the European Union.

It is widely assumed that supportive family members adequately meet the needs of people with dementia from ethnic minorities. However this may not always be the case. Some ethnic groups view dementia as part of normal ageing and are unable to cope properly with a person with dementia's needs. For other groups, dementia and illnesses of the mind are taboo. A study by Dr Richards at the University of London compared small samples of African-Caribbeans and Whites in London. Interviews were conducted including cognitive tests. The main finding was that elderly African-Caribbeans had larger family networks, were more likely to have someone at home with them and were more impaired in activities than Whites. However, there was no evidence to suggest that elderly African-Caribbeans received more help or support from their families anymore that elderly Whites[15].

After establishing the state of research, practice and development in France, the UK and Denmark, the CNEOPSA Project (Care Needs of Minority Ethnic Older Persons Suffering from Alzheimer disease) noted that all three countries commonly share the basic fact that minority ethnic older people are ageing and that they are a permanent settlement in these countries whether their families are with them or not. [15] The project team put forward six recommendations for the care of ethnic minorities with dementia:

Recommendation 1
The following gaps need to be remedied through a planned programme of research and practice developments.

1   Inadequacy of statistics on minority ethnic people with dementia.

2   Figures on the prevalence and the number of persons with dementia are not classified by ethnicity.

3   Information on research, print material and developments in different languages are not available in Denmark and France. Some exist in the UK.

Recommendation 2

The following needs to be considered to improve the situation of minority ethnic older people with dementia and their family carers:

1   A planned information and educational support programme on dementia and care using different modes of communication.

2   A concerted action to improve the socio-economic conditions including improved access to welfare entitlements.

3   Professional care and support to the family carers.

Recommendation 3

It is necessary to build up research, education and training (e.g. skill development) to enable General Practitioners to effectively address the medical problems – within an appropriate cultural, linguistic and anti-discriminatory framework – of minority ethnic older people with dementia.

Recommendation 4

It is essential that appropriate diagnostic instruments are developed and that information to family carers is better explained and communicated.

Recommendations 5

Social and health care professionals are providing an essential service to the care of people with dementia. It is necessary to build up expertise in research, education and training (e.g. skill development) to enable social and health care professionals to provide effective person centred care to minority ethnic older people with dementia, with an appropriate cultural, linguistic, spiritual and anti-discriminatory framework. There is an urgent need to support the development of specialist staff on dementia from minority ethnic groups.

Recommendation 6
There is an urgency to develop specialist resources. A satellite model where investment in a few identified minority ethnic organisations in the UK would be an appropriate step in developing necessary specialist resources. The satellite model could potentially be adapted in Denmark and France where minority ethnic associations do exist but not in the same form as in the UK.

It is always easy to state what should be done but what can be done might be a different story. The phrase 'money makes the world go round' resonates in the minds of policy makers. Can Europe afford adequate provision of dementia care? Some EC- funded projects have addressed this issue.

Economic aspects of dementia
The Karolinska/EACH project looked at the social and economic costs of ADRD and ADRD care[11]. It is pointed out that, as well as an increase in the prevalence of ADRD, Europe may also see a decrease in the proportion of the total population who can provide day to day care and who can pay for the additional care. Recent data from Sweden is provided to illustrate the present situation. Public expenditure for all types of care and nursing for the over 65s has been calculated at 7.37 billion Euro. Cost for people with dementia is estimated at 2.83 billion Euro. This is a great deal of money and is expected to increase. You may well think, no wonder many politicians are turning a blind eye!

However after screening 16,000 scientific journals world-wide for relevant information on the social and economic cost of ADRD, Professor Lennart Levi and the Karolinska/EACH team state that what is needed, both now and in the foreseeable future, is better integration, dissemination and utilisation of existing resources rather than a dramatic increase in funding and staff. Yet again, this comes to the issue of policy. A common European policy is needed to do this. Politicians must not be scared of the cost of adequate dementia care. Long-term thinking today will save money in the future.

The Karolinska/EACH team reviewed many interesting studies relating to this issue. We will look at two studies in particular. The first study is related to Special Care Units (SCUs) which, as we saw in Chapter Six, enhanced the quality of life of patients by reducing behavioural disturbances without resorting to pharmacological or physical restraints. A study in two USA hospitals found that levels of discomfort in SCUs were significantly lower than in a hospital context. The cost over a 3-month period was also lower for the SCU by US$1,500. However the mortality rate amongst people in the SCU was higher than in the traditional care setting (Hurley et al., 1993; Volicer et al., 1994).

Group Living is a care arrangement that can be found in some Member States such as Sweden. A private living arrangement is combined with some form of continuous staffed supervision. Professor Joël and her team at Université Paris Dauphine found that when compared to informal carers who were looking after someone who used expert centres (Belgium), an institution (France), home care (Denmark) or an expert centre (Spain), the informal carers who were looking after someone in a group living situation experienced less subjective 'burden'[16]. However we must not be tempted to conclude from the results of this study that group living involves less 'burden' for carers. Unfortunately, the people these carers were looking after were not matched for severity of dementia. As we saw in Chapter Five, the results from the Middlesex/EACH study showed that the level of disability influenced the carer's stress levels[11]. The results from Paris Dauphine are interesting all the same (especially when considering Wimo et al's finding below) and they merit further research.

Franco Sassi and David McDaid[33] reviewed studies examining the economic aspects of ADRD in the EU. Individual country reports were prepared in 11 European Union countries. Walker (1995) estimated that for all elderly people in Europe two-thirds of care is provided by family members, 13% from the public sector, 11% from the private sector and 3% from voluntary sources. Informal carers incur financial, psychological and social costs. Financial costs are incurred through loss of earnings and through out of pocket expenses in providing for the ADRD sufferers extra care needs. While it is assumed that care in the community reduces costs and that it is in everybody's interests to prolong the time ADRD sufferers can be cared for at home, there are also hidden costs of the additional time in the community as a result of new drug treatments, interventions and supportive services.

Drug treatments
Sassi and McDaid[33] review studies that have evaluated the economic costs and benefits of various treatments and interventions for ADRD patients. Stewart et al (1998) used a five year model to determine the cost per year of life lived with

non-severe dementia for a hypothetical group of patients over the age of 75. The model extrapolated the results of a six-month double blind randomised control trial by Rogers et al (1998) which compared 5mg and 10mg dosages of donepezil with a placebo control. The study concluded that the use of donepezil was almost cost neutral as the savings made in institutional care balanced the drug costs. Another study by Stein (1997) found no clear evidence that donepezil was cost-effective. Similar results were obtained in an Austrian study which analysed the costs and benefits of the drug cerebrolsin.

Living arrangements

In 1991 Wimo et al reported on the cost-effectiveness of group living. It was found that institutional, day care and social service costs were greatly reduced following admission to the group living. However these reductions in cost were offset by the supervision costs of group living. Therefore the average costs per patient per day were not statistically different. However in a later study in 1994, Wimo et al compared the costs of care of a larger group of people with dementia in a group living setting with patients in home care, in day care, and in institutional care. The results showed that the costs of group living were significantly higher than day care or home care for patients at the early stages of dementia. But, the costs of group living did not rise appreciably as the severity of dementia increased, whereas the costs of home care and day care did rise as more intensive forms of care and, in some circumstances, early institutionalisation, had to be introduced to the care package. Wimo et al (1994) concluded that group living might be a less costly alternative than other forms of non-institutional or institutional care when viewed over all stages of dementia progression.

Jozef Pacolet and Ria Bouten reported a study of "Politiques d'aide aux aidants en Europe" at the INSERM conference in Paris[16]. The study analysed the numbers of persons in each Member State receiving residential and day care. Countries oriented towards a Beveridge system of care (Denmark, Sweden, Finland, Norway, Ireland, UK) in the north tended to have higher numbers of both residential and day care service patients per 100 people in the 65 plus age group compared to states oriented towards a Bismarck system in the south, especially the Mediterranean countries. In Flanders Pacolet empirically analysed the time spent by different professionals with AD sufferers living at home. The study was conducted in 1985 and again in 1997. The results are shown in Table 9.1 below.

Table 9.1:   **Time spent by each professional with persons with AD living at home in Flanders, 1985 (550 cases) and 1997 (30 cases)**

	Mins/wk	%	Mins/wk	%
Doctor	11	2.2	11	1.8
Kine	39	7.6	67	11.0
Infirmiere	98	19.2	189	31.1
Aide-senior	338	66.3	302	49.7
Social worker	13	2.5	0.05	0.008
Others	4	0.8	32	5.3
Co-ordination	7	1.4	7	1.1

Using figures of this kind, it is possible to compare the costs of providing care for a person with dementia living at home or living in an institution. Several studies have shown that the costs of institutional care are much higher than care in the family home. Full details of these economic studies can be found by consulting the project reports[11, 16, 33].

The economic imperative

Instead of locking people with dementia away and considering them an annoyance, as was the case fifty years ago, dealing with dementia in a more realistic and person-centred way is now moving up the political agenda. This change of attitude is due to the changing demographic picture of the European population. As a result of falling birth rates and lengthening of life expectancy, the community population is ageing. By 2020 there will 40% more people aged 75 and above than in 1990. This will increase the demand for health services and necessitate changes to their organisation and structure. Over the next 30 years it has been estimated that health care expenditure will increase by at least 1-3% of GDP as a result of these demographic changes. Paying for these increasing costs is made more difficult because the total dependency ratio (the ratio of dependants to workers) is likely to rise from present levels (Communication from the Commission of the European Communities on Development of Public Health Policy in the European Community, Brussels, 15 April, 1998). It has been estimated that by the year 2000, 8 million people in the European Community will be affected by AD alone. There is therefore a strong economic driver behind recent policy developments.

The Maastricht Treaty of 1992 (Article 129, Public health Section) specified the basic competence of the European Community and Member States in the field of health care. The amendments to Article 129 (now Article 152) in the

Amsterdam treaty of 1997 includes "a view to ensuring, and not only contributing to, a high level of human health protection." It can only be hoped that these fine words will be translated into concrete policies and, more importantly, actions to ensure a "high level of human health protection" to the millions of people with dementia and their carers.

Conclusions

Realistic and equitable policies on dementia care need to be introduced in Europe. Health and social services need to work together to improve the implementation of existing policies for people with dementia and their families. There are some key principles on dementia in all Member States that could form the basis of common European policies on dementia care. Once new policies are introduced, commitment and dedication are needed from all concerned to ensure that policies are carried out smoothly. Policies based on long-term thinking will save money in the long run. Appropriate, adequate and accessible care is the right for every person with dementia, no matter what his or her age, culture type of dementia or country of residency.

KEY TERMS

Care in the community

Economic support

Respite care

Equity

CHAPTER 10:   THE FUTURE

As the sun shines through the curtains and announces the break of day Maureen slowly opens her eyes. Unlike her mother who also had Alzheimer's Disease, there is no anxiety as Maureen starts her day. Susan, the community nurse arrives at 9.00 bringing with her the post. More junk mail and special offers from the local gym. Ever since the pop group 'The Graceful Grandees' hit number one with 'Grey Power', there has been an explosion of competition in the service sector. After many years of wise investments and private pensions, the over sixty-fives are considered a lucrative market. It seems strange to think that Maureen's mother and people in her age group were once seen as a burden on society's resources. These days, retired people command respect. Younger people realise their value, not just their monetary value. They are seen as wise and experienced people, people we can learn from. Most organisations and political systems now have a committee of over sixty-fives that they consult about important decisions. Focus groups of the 65-plus group are consulted before every election.

Susan helps Maureen get dressed and they eat breakfast together while listening to Maureen's favourite CDs. Susan knows from her training that familiar music can improve the communication of people with dementia. Susan loves her job. She gets a lot of satisfaction from her constant training and the support from her managers. Around lunchtime, a bus comes to collect Maureen and take her to a nearby school where she and ten other people with dementia have lunch in the school canteen. Wednesday afternoon is music and drama for Year

Five. Maureen and her friends watch and listen as the children stage a show about the 1960s band 'The Beatles'. The children know that they have real expert judges in their audience. They are aware of the nature of their disease and are hoping to bring them some joy and happy memories.

Everybody went home with smiles on their faces; the children proud of their musical talents and the others with an inner happy sensation. When Maureen got home, the house was bustling with familiar sounds. Her grandson was panicking, looking for his football boots, her daughter was shouting at granddaughter for borrowing the car without asking and her son-in-law was entering the house talking to his mobile phone. Some things never change!

A dream perhaps? A fairytale version of dealing with dementia? At the moment, at the turn of the millennium, it would certainly seem so. However the work of the people described in this book is slowly making this lifestyle possible for people with dementia. Where there is a will, there is a way. If we dare to dream, it will happen. What has struck us from writing this book and collating this information is the commitment and enthusiasm of many people working in the field of dementia. As Chapman and Marshall (1996) point out, it is a field that is free from protocol and procedure and imaginative practice is really possible. There are many people who have realised this and are slowly making things happen, changing opinions and bringing new ideas into practice.

This message needs to be spread even further and the will to change things for the better needs to be transmitted to politicians, policy makers and the whole of society. At present, the European Parliament considers ADRD a major health scourge. However this is not the case either at the level of the Council of Ministers or the European Commission. Therefore at the present time there is no specific budget for ADRD and so funding more European projects on dementia care is never guaranteed. However ADRD **is** a health scourge and should never be treated as a normal result of ageing.

Conferences inviting politicians and policy makers are ideal ways to inform and influence these people[1, 2, 4, 11, 21, 22, 23, 32, 33]. Not only do conferences help politicians think about the situation when writing their speeches but they also allow them to mix more closely with people involved in dementia care and to listen to their stories.

The media's role in changing the present situation is very important. The EUROCARE study found that others people's negative reactions to their spouses contributed to their burden [34]. This shows that educating the public more about dementia is necessary. The media could do a lot more to educate the public. In fact, given the right stories, the media could change the ADRD situation overnight. However, at the moment, stories about dementia are not top priority for the media. They are not "sexy" enough. We need imaginative stories from people working in the dementia field to work with the media and to keep feeding stories drip by drip.

Some of the European conferences have produced excellent media coverage. The 5th Alzheimer Europe Annual Meeting in Milan was a good example of how a conference can be successfully run on a low budget and yet stimulate the media. The organiser, Gabriella Salvini Porro, stimulated approximately

80 articles in Italian newspapers about ADRD around the time of the conference[1]. A few conferences have obtained the assistance of a professional PR company. Some of the projects funded by the European Commission have already received plenty of media coverage. Many could still stimulate interest from the media. Box 10.1 below shows a few aspects of projects that could gain media attention.

Box 10.1:   Inviting Media Interest

The 6th Alzheimer Europe Annual Meeting, Warsaw [2]
The fact that this conference was held in Poland created a story in itself. ADRD is a world-wide phenomenon. This conference helped raise awareness in Poland.

Alzheimer Telephone Helpline[3]
Stories on people who have used the helplines.

European Alzheimer's Clearing House (EACH)[4, 11]
General Practitioners' knowledge about ADRD. The high costs of care.

Alzheimer. Un Mal Partagé[6]
'Dailylife' has produced a bank of photographs that correctly portray Alzheimer's Disease. The photographs are very striking and throw a positive light on the disease.

Project for Ambulatory Expertise and Assessment by Expert Centres[7]
Skilled care can comfort patients and their carers.

Te Deum: A Transcultural Educational Dementia project For Europe [12]
The usefulness of information technology to train health care professionals.

Monitoring Neurodegenerative Disease in Europe[14]
The estimates of the magnitude of the problem of ADRD. Estimates of the prognosis of the individuals with the disease.

Handling Alzheimer's Disease in Well Defined Primary health Care of 3 European Distant Regions[20]
Issues related to people with dementia living in rural communities.

Caring for Handicapped People with Dementia An Education Programme[26]
This project brought together carers in order to help them to get to grips with the complexity of problems encountered.

Optimising Support for Informal and Formal Carers of People with Dementia[27]
The importance of and need for early support to both informal and formal carers.

Transnational Analysis of the Socio-economic Impact of Alzheimer's Disease in the European Union[33]
The high costs of formal services and the availability of national and local assistance.

The Alzheimer Associations are already putting a lot of effort into improving the condition of people with ADRD and their families and doing an excellent job in raising public awareness. Alzheimer Europe has produced 'A strategy for the 3rd millennium' which proposes a European awareness campaign. If people involved in the field of ADRD continue to work together, co-operate and aim towards a common goal, then we are on our way to creating a better world for people with ADRD.

together, co-operate and aim towards a common goal, then we are on our way to creating a better world for people with ADRD.

Conclusions

The future for European dementia care could be both exciting and progressive. There are a lot of changes and improvements to be made. To ensure that these happen, policy-makers and the media both have significant roles to play. They are in an excellent position to blaze a trail in making sure that European society deals with dementia effectively. Those who are concerned about dementia must learn to work with these two key groups to enhance public awareness and stimulate positive change. By working together, we can surely find more effective ways of dealing with dementia. Important steps towards this objective are the raising of public awareness and the strengthening of political will. Whatever the factors and concepts that divide society, there is ultimately only one humanity.

Part Three:

EC Project Summaries

CHAPTER 11: ADRD PROJECT SUMMARIES

Part Three summarises the 34 projects that were co-funded by DG V of the European Commission in 1995 and 1996. You will find here for each project the following information:

◆ The project number we have assigned, (1), (2), (3), etc, cited in the above text in superscript form: [1] [2] [3] etc

◆ The project title

◆ The project contract number as assigned by Commission services. These numbers all begin with the three letters "SOC". The next two digits specify the year the contract was awarded, "95" or "96"

◆ The project leader's contact information, should you require further information about the project

◆ Details of other collaborators

◆ The aims and/or objectives of the project

◆ The target group for the project

Following the summary of the thirty-four projects, we conclude with some recommendations concerning the methodology of projects and guidelines for EC project management. We hope that these points will be helpful to applicants for EC funding for projects in the field of dementia.

---

1   The 5th Alzheimer Europe Annual Meeting

Project Contract Number: SOC95 100634

Project Leader's Contact Information
Gabriella Salvini Porro, Federazione Alzheimer Italia,

Via T. Marino 7, 20121 Milano, Italy
TELEPHONE: +39 2 80 97 67
FAX: +39 2 87 57 81
EMAIL: gsalvini@alzheimer.it

Aims and Objectives:

◆ To bring together families and professionals to discuss Alzheimer's Disease.

◆ To promote a debate among Member States between professional, practitioners and researcher in order to foster co-ordination of common guidelines regarding policies and programmes for human health protection and prevention of diseases.

◆ To look at Alzheimer's Disease from an integrated viewpoint.

◆ To consider relevant ethical issues.

Target Group:

Families, Alzheimer's associations and families

Other Collaborators:

The conference was co-sponsored by the World Health Organisation

2   The 6th Alzheimer Europe Annual Meeting, Warsaw

Project Contract Number: SOC95 102970

Project Leader's Contact Information

Jeannot Krecké, Alzheimer Europe, Route de Thionville 145, L2611 Luxembourg.
TELEPHONE: + 352 29 79 70
FAX +352 29 79 72
EMAIL: info@alzheimer-europe.org

Aims and Objectives:
The aim of the conference was to raise the awareness of dementia among specialists, carers and politicians and to learn about and share experiences in caring for the patients and their families

Target Group: Carers and families and professionals

Other Collaborators: Polish Alzheimer's Association

---

3 The Alzheimer Telephone Helpline

Project Contract Number: SOC95 101760

Project Leader's Contact Information
Jeannot Krecké, Alzheimer Europe, Route de Thionville 145, L2611 Luxembourg
TELEPHONE: + 352 29 79 70
FAX: +352 29 79 72
EMAIL: info@alzheimer-europe.org

Aims and Objectives:
To provide a manual for Alzheimer's associations wanting to set up a telephone helpline, or wanting to improve their existing services.

Target Group:
Other Collaborators: Alzheimer Angehorige Austria (Austria), Alzheimer Scotland - Action on Dementia (Scotland), Alzheimer Liga (Belgium), Alzheimer's Disease Society (UK), Alzheimer-Keskuslitto (Finland), Federazione Alzheimer Italia (Italy), Alzheimer Society of Ireland (Ireland), Alzheimerstichting (Netherlands), Fundación Alzheimer España (Spain), Association Luxembourg Alzheimer (Luxembourg).

---

4   EUROPEAN ALZHEIMER CLEARING HOUSE (EACH). This project was funded both in 1995 and 1996.

Project Contract Number: SOC95 102167
(see project[11] below for further details)

---

5   Training, Teaching and Support (T.T.S.) Group for the Alzheimer Programme of the European Commission: A Training Programme for the Carers of People with Dementia

Project Contract Number: SOC95 101761

Project Leader's Contact Information
Overspaarne/Anton Pieck-hofje, Mr. Niek de Boer, Boerhaavelaan 50, 2035 RC Haarlem, Netherlands.
TELEPHONE: +31 23 53 39 108
FAX: +31 23 53 51 744

Other Collaborators:
Marie- Jo Guisset (Fondation de France, France), Dominique Argoud (Cleirppa, France), Pierre-Henri Daure (Fedosad, France), Leny Haaring (Overspaarne, Netherlands), Edith Hanson (Dane Age, Denmark), Palle Pedersen (Odense Kommune, Denmark), Mercé Perez Salanova, (Diputacio de Barcelona, Spain), Karen Margrethe Sorensen (DaneAge, Denmark), Hugo Van waarde (Anton Pieckhofje, Netherlands), Imelda Weir (PSS, United Kingdom), Javier Yanguas Lezaun (Residencia de Eibar/Diputacion foral de Gipuzkoa, Spain), Anne Lise Zilmer (Odense Kommune, Denmark).

Aims and Objectives:
◆   The general task of the T.T.S. group was to develop and

make available to as large a public as possible, programmes and methods for teachings, training and supporting people. The main aim of this project was to exchange and to develop ideas, methods and examples of good practice in the field of teaching, training and supporting people (professionals, family and volunteers) who care for the elderly suffering from Alzheimer's disease and other related disorders.

◆ The second goal was to disseminate these ideas, methods and examples throughout the European Community

Target Group:
Carers of people with Alzheimer's Disease and other related disorders, family, volunteers and professionals.

---

6 Alzheimer. Un Mal Partagé

Project Contract Number: SOC95 10207905

Project Leader's Contact Information
Carl Cordonnier, Dailylife, 34 Rue Louise Michel, 59260 Hellemmes, France
TELEPHONE: +33 3 20 56 18 90
FAX +33 3 20 43 14 76

Aims and Objectives:
To create a bank of photographs on Alzheimer's Disease that are positive and correctly portray Alzheimer's Disease.

Target Group:
Family Associations, Specialists, the Media

Other Collaborators: Dr Florence Lebert, Centre de la Mémoire, Bailleul, France. ADERMA. European Alzheimer's Clearing House. La Féderation Alzheimer Europe Sud. Flandre Alzheimer. L'Association des

Journalists Européens. L'Institut de Bioéthique de Maastricht. Le Centre Médical des Monts de Flandre

---

7 Project for Ambulatory Expertise and Assessment by Expert Centres

Project Contract Number: SOC95 101973

Project Leader's Contact Information
Professeur R. Moulias, Société Française de Gérontologie, 105 boulevard de l'hôpital, 75013 Paris, France
FAX: +33 1 40 77 96 44.
EMAIL: robert.moulias@cfx.ap-hop-paris.fr

Aims and Objectives:
To know the typology of the centres, diagnosis procedures, therapeutic procedures (including drugs, new drugs, psychological and social care), networks, place in training and research, especially family carer training in the different countries

Target Group: Elderly patients

Other Collaborators:
32 Alzheimer expertise centres in 15 European countries.

---

8 Qualité de Vie. Formation et Assistance des Familles

Project Contract Number: SOC95 101949

Project Leader's Contact Information
Roland Lamontagne and Mychele Beuchat, Fédération Association Alzheimer Su-Europe (FASE), 3 Avenue des Palmiers, F6600 Perpignan, France
TELEPHONE/ FAX:+33 68 35 796

Aims and Objectives:
To increase the quality of life of people with Alzheimer's Disease by helping their carers to better understand Alzheimer's and optimise the capacities of the person with Alzheimer's Disease

Target Group: Family and professional carers

Other Collaborators:
L'AFAC de Barcelone, L'Université de Gerone, L'Hôpital de Perpignan, Espiral Serveis Als Grans

---

9   European Self-Help Carer Manual

Project Contract Number: SOC96 202 090

Project Leader's Contact Information
Jeannot Krecké, Alzheimer Europe, Route de Thionville 145, L2611 Luxembourg.
TELEPHONE: + 352 29 79 70
FAX: +352 29 79 72
EMAIL: info@alzheimer-europe.org

Aims and Objectives:
To increase the quality of life of people with Alzheimer's Disease by helping their carers to better understand Alzheimer's and optimise the capacities of the person with Alzheimer's Disease

Target Group: Family and professional carers

Other Collaborators:
Gabriella Salvini, Italy. Ruth Clausen, Denmark. Irene Smoor, Netherlands. Camilla Goetschalckx, Luxembourg. Antonia Croy, Austria. Henriette Chamouillet, DGV,

European Commission. Leena Kulju, Finland. Norman Stuart, Ireland. Harry Cayton, England. Jacques Selmes, Spain. Jean Georges, Alzheimer Europe. Dianne Gove, Alzheimer Europe. Marie-Laure Tortel, Alzheimer Europe

---

10 Bureau Européen pour l'information et la Co-ordination Alzheimer

Project Contract Number: SOC96 201162

Project Leader's Contact Information

Jeannot Krecké, Alzheimer Europe,
Route de Thionville 145, L2611 Luxembourg
TELEPHONE: + 352 29 79 70
FAX: +352 29 79 72
EMAIL: info@alzheimer-europe.org

Aims and Objectives:

◆ The co-ordination of the setting up of organisations in countries and regions with limited facilities.

◆ The co-ordination of relations between countries of the European Economic Area and Eastern European countries.

◆ The role of intermediary between the different European associations in view of the setting up and co-ordination of common and transnational projects.

◆ The setting up of an inventory of existing European organisations operating in the field of Alzheimer's disease and related disorders with regard to their structure, services and mode of financing.

◆ The collection of information and statistical data on projects and relevant models already available in Europe and other countries and this in collaboration with Alzheimer's Disease International.

◆ Arrangement for the translation of texts of general interest in the field of Alzheimer's disease and related problems.

◆ The carrying out of preparatory work in view of the setting up a computer network, which will, on the one hand, assemble the associations active in the field of Alzheimer's disease and, on the other hand, be used to distribute the information via the internet to the general public, professional, political and administrative bodies.

Target Group:
Alzheimer's Associations and the general public

Other Collaborators:
European Alzheimer's Associations

---

11 EUROPEAN ALZHEIMER CLEARING HOUSE (EACH). This project was funded both in 1995 and 1996

Project Contract Number: SOC95 102167

Project Leader's Contact Information
Professor Franz Baro, EACH, c/o Esplanade Building - Room 303, 19 B5, 1010 Brussels - Belgium
TELEPHONE: +32 2 210 44 62
FAX: +32 2 210 44 62
EMAIL:EACH@Health.fgov.be

Aims and Objectives:
◆ EACH aims to make better use of existing information and expertise of good practice in the field of care for patients with Alzheimer's Disease and related disorders. The project puts forward a number of aspects of high importance for patients and carers, especially in ADRD care but also in public health

in general. The selected priority projects are Training, Good Practice, Alzheimer Associations, Socio-Economic Impact, Ethical Issues, Support Programmes, Nursing Qualifications, Substance Counselling, Clinical Specifics.

◆ The objective of EACH is to collect, analyse, compile, disseminate and promote the application of the knowledge about different aspects of ADRD and its consequences, the optimal ways of management for patients, their families, caregivers, administrators, decision makers and the general public, the knowledge-based care to achieve the highest possible level of living and quality of life for patients and their families.

The overall aim is to contribute substantially in the field of information, education and policy development in favour of persons suffering of ADRD in order to improve public awareness, services, quality of life for patients and their families, empowerment of self help, policy development and the common core of cultural specifics between European countries.

Target Group:

People with Alzheimer's Disease and Related Disorders, their family, non-professional and professional caregivers, self-help movements, educators, administrators, decision makers and the public at large

Other Collaborators:

Environment (Brussels-BE), Alzheimer Europe (Luxembourg-LU), Fundacion Alzheimer España (Madrid-ES), European Medical Association (Brussels-BE), Jewish Care (London-UK), Dementia Services Development Centre (Stirling-Scotland), National Swedish Institute for

Psychosocial Factors and Health (Stockholm-SE), Higher Institute of Labour Studies (Leuven-BE), Institute for Bioethics (Maastricht-NL), Belgian Inter-university Centre for Research Action on Health and Psychosocial Factors (Bierbeek-BE) Health Research Centre - Middlesex University (London-UK), Council for Health and Social Service (Zoetermeer-NL), University of Rennes - Dept of Clinical Pharmacology (Rennes-FR), Acute Stroke Advisory Panel (Stuttgar-GE), University of Antwerp, Dept Neurochemistry and Behaviour (Antwerp-BE).

12 Te Deum: A Transcultural Educational Dementia Project For Europe

Project Contract Number: SOC96 202088

Project Leader's Contact Information

Professor Dr Heyrman, Academisch Centrum Huisartsgeneeskunde, Kapucijnenvoer 33 blok J, b 3000 Leuven, Belgium.
TELEPHONE: +32 16 33 74 68
FAX: +32 16 33 74 80
EMAIL: Jan.Heyrman@med.kuleuven.ac.be

Aims and Objectives:

To measure the didactic qualities of an interactive computer based training programme for General Practitioners to improve diagnosis of dementia and to look for the needed adaptations for distribution in other countries.

Target Group:

General Practitioners in the Netherlands, UK and France

Other Collaborators:

Dr J Degryse and Dr J De Lepeleire, Katholieke Universiteit

Leuven, Professor L. Southgate, University College London. Dr B.Gay, College National des Généralistes Enseignants. Dr M. Vernooij, Universiteit Nijmegen.

13 Coping with Alzheimer Type Dementia in Older People with Intellectual Disability

Project Contract Number: SOC96 202151

Project Leader's Contact Information
Nancy Breitenbach c/o Inclusion International, 13D Chemin du Levant, 01210, Ferney-Voltaire, France or Jean-Marc Faure, Retroviseur, 38480 St Martin De Vaulserre, France

Aims and Objectives:
To produce a video documentary and brochure on the issue of dementia in older people with life-long intellectual disability.

Target Group: Informal and formal carers. The general public

Other Collaborators:
Dr Henry van Schrojenstein Lantman de Valk, Pepijn Centre, The Netherlands. Dr Marian Maaskant, Pepijn Centre, The Netherlands. Harry Urlings, Pepijn Centre, The Netherlands. Jacky Vandevelde, APEMH, Luxembourg. Dr Germain Weber, Insitut für Psychologie der Universität, Austria. Steve Moss, University of Manchester, UK. Lars Molander, Sweden

14 Monitoring Neurodegenerative Diseases in Europe

Project Contract Number: SOC96 202098

Project Leader's Contact Information
Prof. A. Hofman, Dr LJ Launer, Dept of Epidemiology and Biostatistics, Erasmus University Medical School, PO Box

1738, Rotterdam, the Netherlands
TELEPHONE: +31-10-408-7488
FAX: +31-10-408-5933
EMAIL: hofman@epib.fgg.eur.nl

Aims and Objectives:

The general objective of the collaborative network is to monitor the magnitude of the problem of neurodegenerative diseases in older persons living in the European Community. The specific objectives are to:

♦ Monitor the prevalence of neurodegenerative diseases dementia (sub-types), Parkinson's disease and stroke) in Europe to provide an estimate of the magnitude of the problem;

♦ Monitor the incidence of neurodegenerative diseases to provide an estimate of individual risk;

♦ Study the prognosis of individuals with neurodegenerative diseases.

Target Group:

Health planners and researchers in the field of neurologic diseases of the elderly.

Other Collaborators:

Dr K. Andersen, Odense Hospital, Denmark. Dr K. Berger, Wilhelms University, Germany. Dr M.M.B. Breteler, Erasmus University Rotterdam, The Netherlands. Professor Copeland, University of Liverpool, UK. Professor J.F. Dartigues, University Bordeaux II, France. Dr A. Di Carlo, Area della Ricerca di Firenze, Italy. Dr L. Fratiglioni, Stockholm Gerontology Research Centre, Sweden. Dr C. Jagger, University of Leicester, UK. Professor A. Lobo Clínica Universitaria Zaragoza, Spain.

Professor J.M. Martinez Lage and Dr J.M. Manubens, Universidad de Navarra, Spain. Dr M. De Rijk, Erasmus University Rotterdam, The Netherlands. Dr R. Schmidt, Karl Franzens University Gaz, Austria. Professor H. Soininen, Kuopio University, Finland.

---

15 CNEOPSA: Meeting Care Needs of Minority Ethnic Older Persons Suffering from Alzheimer's Disease

Project Contract Number: SOC96 38074

Project Leader's Contact Information

Content: Naina Patel, Management Centre, Bradford University, Emm Lane Bradford, BD9 4JL,UK.
TELEPHONE: +44 113 294 7189
FAX: +44 113 295 8221
EMAIL: N.Patel5@bradford.ac.uk

Administration: Omar Samaol, OGMF, Hôpital Paul Brousse F - 94804, VILLEJUIF, France
TELEPHONE: +33 1 45 59 31 30
FAX: +33 145 59 39 45

Aims and Objectives:

◆ To establish Country Profiles for UK, Denmark and France.

◆ To inform and increase awareness on dementia care to minority ethnic older people among key groups in each country.

◆ To generate culturally appropriate knowledge and practice through a guide on Good Practice (see Examples of Good Practice).

◆ To exchange knowledge, findings and analysis via seminar held in each country.

◆ To promote the area generally as an urgent one requiring planned action.

Target Group:
Policymakers, Researchers, Dementia specific and Minority organisations, Carers Trainers

Other Collaborators:
Peter Lindblad, Danish Institute of Gerontology, Denmark

---

16 Conditions of Caregivers in Charge of Patients with Dementia of the Alzheimer Type. Economic Analysis of the Impact of the Different Care Management Systems

Project Contract Number: SOC96 202257

Project Leader's Contact Information
Dr Marie-Eve Joël, Laboratoire d'Economie et de Gestion des Organisations de Santé, Université Paris-Dauphine, Place du Maréchal de Lattre de Tassigny, 75775 Paris, Cedex 16.
TELEPHONE: +33 1 44 05 45 18
FAX: +33 1 44 05 41 27
EMAIL: joel@dauphine.fr

Aims and Objectives:
◆ The objective of this research is to analyse - comparatively and at the European level - the condition of informal caregivers in charge of patients with dementia of the Alzheimer type.

◆ To find out the impact of the various systems of care management in economic terms as well as on their quality of life.

♦ To compare six different types of care management for those in Europe who are suffering from Alzheimer's disease or related disorders (Home Care (Denmark), Expert Centre (Spain), Institution (France), Day Centre (Germany), Group Living (Sweden) and Expert Centre (Belgium). The common characteristic of these programmes is to organise care management co-ordinated to the patient and his primary informal caregiver.

Target Group:
The caregivers of patients with dementia of the Alzheimer type as part of six care programs.

Other Collaborators:
Laboratoire d'Economie et de Gestion des Organisations de Santé: Dr Agnès Gramain, Mme Elisabeth Cozette, Mlle Caroline Grisard, Dr Isabelle Vedel, Mlle Béatrice Guillebaud, Mlle Elodie Bertand.

Associated research team in the Unit 500 of the Institut National pour la Santé et la Recherche Médicale: Dr Alain Colvez, Dr Anne-Charlotte Royer, Mlle Sophie Bardel.

---

17 Comparative Analysis of Socio-Medical Assistance Systems for Aged People Attacked by Neurodegenerating Diseases (Alzheimer especially), In Order to Promote Training Aimed for Home Care Providers

Project Contract Number: SOC96 202 154

Project Leader's Contact Information
Christine Flori, Services Emploi Dévelopment Initiatives (SEDI), 37, rue de Nantes 75019 PARIS, France.

TELEPHONE: +33 1 42 05 37 86
FAX: +33 1 40 35 25 77

Other Collaborators:
FRANCE: Professor Robert Moulias , Hôpital Charles
Foix. Jean Biarnes, Université Paris XIII.M. Michel
Aberlen, Délégation Nationale à l' Emploi et à la
Formation Professionnelle. Marie Santiago Delefosse,
Chercheur CNRS (équipe 1478). Albert Azoulay,
Université Paris XIIII. Christian Ballouard, Laboratoire
d'Ethique Médicale, Hôpital Necker, Paris. AUSTRIA:
M. Klaus Besselmann , Kuratorium Deutsche Altershilfe.
UK: M. Andrew Fairbairn - Newcastle City Health,
Headquarters. ITALY: Mme Patrizia Spadin, AIMA.
LUXEMBOURG: M. Lars Rasmussen, Commission des
Communautés Européennes. PORTUGAL: Mme Dr.
Quintela, Ministerio do Emprego e da segurança social.
SWEDEN: Mme Britt Mari Hellner, Socialstyrelsen.

Aims
◆ To update knowledge on the ways and means of
providing care for elderly people suffering from
neurodegenerative disorders especially Alzheimer's.

◆ Foster new discussions and exchanges, at the European
level, on the expertise required to provide care for the
patients under consideration and to ensure that home care
services are efficient and of a high standard.

◆ Continuation of the work of the Société Française de
Gérontologie (Prof. Moulias) which assessed the provision of
care by Expert Centres for the patients under consideration
and drew up recommendations on home care for such
patients. This project is a logical follow-up of the provision of

home care services since its aim is to propose an organisation of these services and training for care providers.

Objectives:

◆ To become acquainted with and assess the needs of these patients and of their immediate circle (family, entourage, professional care providers).

◆ To compare the medical-social systems in the six countries selected.

◆ To propose suitable training schemes for home care providers and to help promote these training schemes, particularly with training institutions and instructors.

Target Group: Informal and Formal Carers

---

18 Early Diagnosis of Vascular Dementia, Validated Criteria, Clinical/MRI Features, and Risk Factors of Vascular Cognitive Impairment (VCI)

Project Contract Number: SOC96 202167

Project Leader's Contact Information
Dr Pablo Martinez-Lage, Hospital Virgen Del Camino, Irunlarrea, 4, 31008 Pamplona, Spain
TELEPHONE: +34 948 42 94 00
FAX: +34 948 17 05 15

Other Collaborators:
Dr Jose Manubens, Spain. Dr John Bowler, London

Aims and Objectives:
To define the neurological criteria of people who have mild cognitive impairment of vascular origin

Target Group:
>   People who have had a stroke or have vascular risk factors

---

19 The Special Care Unit for Demented Persons in Nursing Home: A Case Control Study on Efficacy in the Improvement of Quality of Life of Patients and their Relatives

Project Contract Number: SOC96 202 171

Project Leader's Contact Information
>   Dr Giovanni Frisoni, Alzheimer's Unit, IRCCS, San Giovanni - FBF, Via Pilastroni 1, 25123, Brescia , Italy

Aims and Objectives:
>   To assess the effect of specialised institutional care on behaviourally disturbed patients with dementia.

Target Group:
>   People with dementia and behavioural disturbances, and their carers

Other Collaborators:
>   Professor Bengt Winblad and Professor Laura Fratiglioni, Sweden. Bruno Vellas, France. Marco Trabucchi and Angelo Bianchetti, Italy

---

20 Handling Alzheimer's Disease in Well Defined Primary Health Care Area of 3 European Distant Regions

Project Contract Number: SOC96 202236 05F03

Project Leader's Contact Information
>   Ass. Prof. Christos Lionis, Department of Social Medicine, P.O. Box 1393, Heraklion, Crete, Greece.

TELEPHONE: +30 81 394 621
FAX: +30 81 394 606
EMAIL: lionis@fortezza.cc.ucr.gr

Aims and Objectives:

◆ To access the level of knowledge of neurodegenerative disease, particularly DAT of primary health care (PHC) workers (medical doctors, district nurses and social workers) who are functioning in a number of health centres in well-defined areas of Crete, Greece, Ostergotland, Sweden and Iceland. To develop training for carers, as well as to develop manuals and other educational tools.

◆ To estimate the number of aged people who suffer from DAT in these well-defined areas and the use of PHC and hospital services for these patients.

◆ To determine the social , psychological and economical impact of the disease on their families in Crete.

◆ To inform local authorities, particularly staff of municipalities and country councils of the different aspects of Alzheimer's disease and related disorders in Crete.

Target Group:

Primary health care providers working in well-defined areas in three European regions. People living in rural Crete who have dementia but have not been diagnosed

Other Collaborators:

Professor Erik Trell, University of Linkoping, Sweden.
Dr Kristajanson Ingolfur, Reykjvik, Iceland.

21 European Conference on Alzheimer's Disease and Related Disorders

Project Contract Number: SOC96 201802

Project Leader's Contact Information
Susan Riley, Department of Health Hawkins House, Dublin, Ireland

Aims and Objectives:
To bring together professionals from different fields working on ADRD Projects

Target Group: Professionals working on ADRD

Other Collaborators: Alzheimer Society Ireland

---

22 The Second European Congress on Nutrition and Health in the Elderly

Project Contract Number: SOC96 200941

Project Leader's Contact Information
Marianne Schroll, Department of Geriatrics HL, Kommunehospitalet, Oster Farimagsgade 5, DK-1399 Kobenhavn K., Denmark
TELEPHONE +45 33 38 36 45
FAX +45 33 38 36 69

Aims and Objectives:
- To increase the understanding, prevention and treatment of nutritional problems in the elderly, especially those suffering from Alzheimer's disease and related disorders.
- To strengthen the quality of methods to be used in nutritional surveys and clinical geriatric medicine.

- ◆ To further the propagation of results from nutrition research in the elderly, especially those suffering from Alzheimer's disease and related disorders.

- ◆ To develop professional networks in Europe

Target Group:
Researchers in Nutrition and Health in the Elderly in Europe

Other Collaborators:
Carsten Hendriksen, Dept. of Geriatrics HL, Kommunehospitalet, Oster Farimagsgade 5, 1399 Kobenhavn, Denmark

---

23 The 13th International Conference on Alzheimer's Disease International and 7th Annual Meeting of Alzheimer Europe: "Alzheimer's - The Blind Hunter", September 29- October 1, 1997, Helsinki, Finland

Project Contract Number: SOC96 202246

Project Leader's Contact Information

Alzheimer Society of Finland & Executive Director Ms. Varpu Kettunen, Luosikatu 4E, Fin-00160 Helsinki.
TELEPHONE: +358-9-6226 200
FAX: +358-9-6226 2020
EMAIL: varpu.kettunen@alzheimer.fi

Aims and Objectives:
To provide a unique opportunity for scientists, nursing personnel as well as caregivers affected with dementia to share and receive support, strength and knowledge of the latest developments in the field. The intention

was to create an informal, highly stimulating atmosphere for fruitful discussions and networking.

Target Group:
Professional working in the field of dementia, carers, journalists, policy makers

Other Collaborators:
Alzheimer's Disease International and Alzheimer Europe

24 The Equal Project: Enhancing the Quality of Life of Older People with Alzheimer's disease

Project Contract Number: SOC96 20209505

Project Leader's Contact Information
Ms. B. Penhale, Social Work Department, University of Hull, Kingston Upon Hull HU6 7RX
TELEPHONE: 01482 465716
FAX: 01482 466306
EMAIL: B.L.PENHALE@comhealth.hull.ac.uk

Aims and Objectives:
- To produce a template of best practice in the development of reminiscence groups for older people with Alzheimer's disease which are transferable cross-culturally.
- To promote the development of volunteers' skills.
- To increase involvement and of groups within their local communities.
- To enhance quality of life of older people with Alzheimer's disease through innovatory, intergenerational reminiscence projects.

Target Group:
People with Alzheimer's Disease

Other Collaborators:

Three co-participants in Hull: Bradley, Parker and Manthorpe.
Two partners: Sweden (Vaxjo) and France (Marseille)

---

25 The Use of Small Housing Units for Persons with Dementia

Project Contract Number: SOC96 202233

Project Leader's Contact Information

Marie-Jo Guisset, Fondation de France, 40 Avenue
Hoche, 75008 Paris, France
TELEPHONE: +33 1 44 21 31 30

Aims and Objectives:

To analyse ways in which small housing units can be
adapted in every respect to offer flexible and personal
care in the community to dementia sufferers. In
particular, it was examined:

◆ whether the current work in small units shows that these
are suitable for people suffering from dementia.

◆ what conditions are necessary to improve the current
work in small units with respect to the needs of the
people suffering from dementia, in particular in the areas
of (a) architecture and use of space, (b) organisation of
day to day life (c) finance and management
arrangements, (d) the combination of formal and informal
care, including the involvement of families.

Target Group: People with dementia

Other Collaborators:

Projects of the Salmon Group in Spain, France, Belgium,
Holland, Germany and the UK. Dr Kai Leichsenring,
European Centre, Vienna

26 Caring for the Dementia-Handicapped Patient - An Education Programme

Project Contract Number: SOC96 202200

Project Leader's Contact Information

Associate Professor Gertrud Grahn, PhD Kurland 55 SE-231 93 Trelleborg Sweden.
TELEPHONE/FAX: +46 410 33 09 39

Contact Information:

Professor Barbo Beck-Friis, MD PhD, Silviahemmet, Box 142 SE-178 02 Drottningholm, Sweden
TELEPHONE: +46 8 759 00 71
FAX: +46 8 759 00 74

Aims and Objectives:

To test an education programme (including learning materials) named 'Living with Dementia' developed to enable health care professional and relatives caring for dementia-handicapped people to create optimal conditions regarding the patients' functioning and well being and to assure dignity for the dementia-handicapped patient.

Target Group:

Health care professionals and relatives caring for people with dementia

Other Collaborators:

Stiftelsen Silviahemmet, Sweden and Professor Beck-Friis, MD, PhD

27 Optimising Support for Informal and Formal Carers of People with Dementia

Project Contract Number: SOC96 202176

Project Leader's Contact Information

Annika Sundkler, City District of Orgryte, Elderly Care, Box 6244, 400 60 GOTEBORG, Sweden.
TELEPHONE: +46 31 852400
FAX: +46 31 84793
EMAIL: annica.sundkler@orgryte.goteborg.se

Other Collaborators:

Portugal: Dr Antonio Leuschner, Hospital Magalhaes Lemos. Ireland: Maureen Caffrey, North Eastern Health Board, Navan. Northern Ireland: Marie Heaney, South and East Belfast Trust, Belfast

Aim:

To enable elderly people with dementia to remain safely in their home settings by optimising informal and formal care.

Objectives

♦ To identify the support information and skill needs of informal carers.

♦ To develop appropriate responses to the identified needs.

♦ To develop a competency based training package for formal carers.

♦ To explore the area of risk assessment and management in home care of people with dementia.

Target Group:

Elderly suffering from dementia and their carers, formal and informal

28 Individualised Memory Aids for Persons with Alzheimer-Type Dementia

Project Contract Number: SOC96 202190

Project Leader's Contact Information

Dr Fred Furniss, Centre for Applied Psychology, University of Leicester, LE1 7RH.
TELEPHONE: +44 116 252 2480
FAX: +44 116 252 2503
EMAIL: fred.furniss@leicester.ac.uk

Aims and Objectives:

Bourgeois (1990, 1992, 1993) has shown that use of simple memory aids enhances the quality of conversation of persons with Alzheimer-type dementia. The aim was to replicate Bourgeois' intervention with five persons with severe dementia (Mini-Mental State Examination scores 0-12) and diagnoses of Alzheimer-type, multi-infarct or vascular dementia, and evaluated the impact of the aids on the proportion of time participants spent on topic in conversation with carers.

Target Group:

People with severe Alzheimer-type dementia

Other Collaborators:

Dr. C. Sdogati, COO.S.S. Marche. Italy

29 Health Promoting Intervention for Alzheimer's Family Caregivers. Development of a Training Programme to Improve Individual and Social Resources

Project Contract Number: SOC96 202103

Project Leader's Contact Information

Prof. Klaus Klein, University of Cologne, Faculty of Education, Health Education Research Unit, Gronewaldstr. 2, D-50931 Koln, Germany
TELEPHONE: +49 221 470 4652
FAX: +49 221 470 5174
EMAIL: Klein@ew.uni-koeln.de

Aims and Objectives:

◆ Development of culturally appropriate European training program that provides advice, support and answers to problems of Alzheimer's family caregivers taking into account the psychological dimension of the disease.

◆ Improvement of self-help potentials according to the concept of health promotion: healthy behaviour should be incorporated into the daily living and thus the quality of life of patients and caregivers should be increased.

◆ Definition of deficits and gaps as well as potentials in the psychosocial and nursing care of Alzheimer's disease in participating member states.

◆ Preparation of a report on the psychological support for Alzheimer's private caregivers.

◆ Analysis of the relations between patients and caregivers in order to identify problems and needs.

◆ Evaluation and dissemination of training package in participating countries.

◆ improvement of national Alzheimer Associations.

Target Group:

Target groups for the training program are counsellors/skilled personnel (professional and non-professional) in self-help organisations and social, health care and other institutions providing support for private caregivers

Other Collaborators:

Germany: Dr. Michael Apel, Christine Max, Patricia Roser, Martina Humbach, Cara Pauls.

Participants:

Prof. Ilse Krypsin-Exner, Psychology, University of Vienna, Austria. Prof. Alain Deccache, Health Education, Univerite Catholique de Louvain, Belgium. Dr. Christine Swane, Sociologist, Danish Institute of Gerontology, Denmark. Prof. Raimo Sulkava, Geriatrician, University of Kyopio, Finland. Jean Michel Rossignol, Secretary General of "Foundation Nationale De Gerontologie", France. Prof. Klaus Klein, Educationalist, Health Education Research Unit, Germany. Sara Turner, Clinical Psychologist, Pathfinder Mental Health Services NHS Trust, Great Britain. Prof. Yannis Skalkidis, MD, Health Education, Hellenic Society for Quality in Health Care, Greece. Brian Neeson, Health Promotion Officer, Mid Western Health board, Ireland. Prof. Fabrizio Fabris, Geriatrician, University of Torino, Italy. Camilla Gittschalckx, Educationalist, Association Luxembourg Alzheimer, Luxemburg. Leonne Groenewegen, Educationalist, Aquest Consultory LTD, Netherlands. Dr. Olivia Robusto Leitao, MD, Alzheimer Association Portugal, Portugal. Prof. Miquel Aguilar Barbera, Neurologist, Hospital Mutua de Terrassa, Spain. Prof. Urban Rosenqvist, MD, Health Education, University of Uppsala, Sweden.

30 Transnational European Analysis of Public Health Policy Developments For Alzheimer's and Associated Disorders of Elderly People and their Carers

Project Contract Number: SOC 96202086

Project Leader's Contact Information
Professor Morton Warner, Welsh Institute for Health and Social Care, University of Glamorgan, Pontypridd CF37 1DL
TELEPHONE: +44 1443 48 30 70
FAX: +44 1443 483079
EMAIL: mlongley@glam.ac.uk

Aims and Objectives:

◆ To examine working definitions of cognitive impairment across Europe and to demonstrate the clinical, social and legal implications of these definitions.

◆ To investigate the relationships of these definitions with policy and practice across Europe.

◆ To pinpoint landmarks in the disease process (indicating the need for a decision about whether to intervene) across European nations.

◆ To explore the factors associated with cognitive impairment and the identification of Alzheimer's Disease, including how health and social gains are measured e.g. the clinical detection of memory impairment and/or a breakdown in the capacity to cope, and the support networks available to women, in particular, as carers.

Target Group:
Policy makers at the national and health service delivery levels.

Other Collaborators:
Professor Sally Furnish, University of Manchester.
Professor Brian Lawlor, Trinity College, Dublin

---

31 Transmural Intervention in Problems with Dementia at Home: A Randomised Controlled Study (Alzheimer)

Project Contract Number: SOC96 202197

Project Leader's Contact Information
Professor Meindert Haveman, The Institute for
Psychosocial and Epidemiological Research (IPSER),
Postbus 214, NL – 6200 AE Maastricht, The Netherlands
TELEPHONE: +31 43 32.99.773
FAX: +31 43 32 99.708

Aims and Objectives:
To test and evaluate the implementation of a comprehensive transmural programme in the homecare for patients with dementia as a first stage for structural implementation of the programme in the regions.

Target Group:
Those who organise services to support informal carers

Other Collaborators:
René Reijnders, (IPSER). Servei Catala de la Salut, Barcelona and Terrassa, Spain; Regional Centre for Ambulatory Mental Health Care Maastricht, Dept. of Senior Citizen Services, The Netherlands; University Psychiatric Centre, St Kamillus, Bierbeek, Belgium.

32 Widening Horizons in Dementia

Project Contract Number: SOC96 202101

Project Leader's Contact Information

Pam Schweitzer, Age Exchange Reminiscence Centre, 11 Blackhealth Village, London, SE3 G LA

TELEPHONE: +44 181 318 9105

FAX: +44 318 0060

EMAIL: age-exchange@lewisham.gov.uk

Aims and Objectives:

◆ To promote imaginative approaches to improving the quality of life of people with dementia and those who care for them.

◆ To highlight the value of reminiscence as a way of advancing this.

◆ To bring together experts from the fields of social work, medicine, community care and the arts to share experience and pool expertise across European countries.

Target Group: Those who organise dementia care

Other Collaborators:

Angelilca Trilling, Social Services, Kasssel, Germany. Professor Faith Gibson, Ulster University. Margaret Health, Alzheimer's Disease Society, Lewisham, London. Lotta Isas, Ersta Diaconijallkap, Stockholm.

33 Transnational Analysis of the Socio-Economic Impact of Alzheimer's Disease in the European Union

Project Contract Number: SOC96 202099

Project Leader's Contact Information

Mr Franco Sassi, LSE Health, London School of Economics and Political Science, Houghton Street, London, WC2A 2AE
TELEPHONE: +44 171 955 7566
FAX: + 44 171 955 6803
EMAIL: sassi@lse.ac.uk

Aims and Objectives:

♦   To improve the understanding of the social and economic issues related to the provision of formal and informal care to people with dementia of the Alzheimer type.

♦   To facilitate the circulation of ideas between members states and disseminate best practice.

♦   To describe the patterns of AD, and the organisational and financing models of care currently adopted in 11 EU Member States.(Exceptions are Greece, Ireland, Belgium and Luxembourg).

♦   To analyse resource implications of AD related to health and social services provided by both the formal and informal sectors.

♦   To measure empirically the social and economic burden borne by families and other informal caregivers in selected EU Member States (UK, Italy and Sweden). The study focused on the impact of providing care to persons with AD, in terms of quality of life, utilisation of health services, employment status, social relationships, and cash expenditures.

Target Group:

Health and social care policy makers and resource managers at all levels responsible for services for people with dementia and the carers throughout Europe are the primary target group. In addition the project should be of great importance to caregivers and their families, as well as the general public and dementia related professionals

Other Collaborators:

Research Centres: Personal Social Services Research Unit - London School of Economics and Political Science. Stockholm Gerontology Centre, Karolinska Institute - Stockholm, Sweden. CERGAS, Universita 'L Bocconi, Milano, Italy. Institut Ostereichische Akademie der Wissenschaften, Wien, Austria. Danish Hospital Institute, Kobenhaven, Denmark. Department of Health Policy and Management, University of Kuopio, Finland. CREDES, Paris, France. University of Hannover, Hannover, Germany. Institute for Medical Technology Assessment, Erasmus University, Rotterdam, The Netherlands. Escola Nacional de Saude Publica, Lisboa, Portugal. Pompeu Fabra University, Barcelona, Spain.

Alzheimer Associations:

Alzheimer Angehoerige Osterreich, Wien, Austria. Alzheimer Society of Finland. Deutsche Alzheimer Gesellschaft, Germany. Federazione Alzheimer Italia, Milano, Italy. Alzheimerstichting, Bunnik, The Netherlands. APFADA, Lisboa, Portugal. Fundacion Alzheimer Espana, Madrid, Spain. Fundacio ACE , Barcelona, Spain.

---

34 The Experience of Spouses Caring for Older People with Dementia of the Alzheimer's Type

Project Contract Number: SOC96 202155

Project Leader's Contact Information

Joanna Murray, Section of Epidemiology and General Practice, Institute of Psychiatry Park, London SE5 8AF.
TELEPHONE: +44 171 919 3126
EMAIL: spjujom@ iop.bpmf.ac.uk

Aims and Objectives:

◆ This was an exploratory study to help clarify the role of different systems of funding health care and social structures on carers' ability and motivation to adopt the role.

◆ To develop hypotheses (the Stress Process Model of Perlin et al., 1990 on factors associated with carer burden and psychological disorders).

Target Group:

Spouses caring for an older person with dementia of the Alzheimer's type in all 15 EC member states.

Other Collaborators:

Justine Schneider, Sube Banerjee, Anthony Mann. (Collaborators in 14 other member states)

CHAPTER 12: THE EUROPEAN COMMISSION'S ADRD PROJECTS: METHODOLOGY, MANAGEMENT AND FUTURE PROSPECTS

Reviewing, summarising and synthesising the EC DG V ADRD projects has been an interesting and challenging task. Some projects have produced a huge amount of new and much needed work in a short timescale. Others have not been so impressive. The limited and fluctuating budget has varied dramatically from year to year and projects have been funded for a single year at a time. Project leaders have therefore designed projects that are intended to last for only one year. For many types of projects, this is too short a period for the projects to be satisfactorily completed from beginning to end. This has meant that project leaders have been forced to produce conclusions based on small–scale studies or on a very small numbers of participants. However projects should not really be attempted or funded unless the aims and objectives are feasible, the methods are sound and the project is to be efficiently co-ordinated and managed.

The fact that these projects are being carried out at a European level is sending an important signal to informal carers, health professionals and all people involved in Alzheimer's Disease and Related Disorders. It shows that they are not alone in dealing with dementia, that ADRD is something that the whole of the European Union is facing and searching for better ways to cope, that people in authority recognise and care about the issue and that the political world is showing an interest. They also have the potential to add a transnational dimension to projects allowing the transfer of good practice, training and information across the Member States. However there is a need for this signal to be amplified, for the message to be much clearer, and the efforts of the Commission in the dementia field to be magnified.

These 34 EC projects have facilitated transnational research and collaboration. The EC Alzheimer's funding has enabled many people to meet, collaborate and share experiences from all over the European Union. There has been exchange and transfer of knowledge, skills and expertise across regions and countries. This would not have happened to the same extent without the participation and financial support of the European Community. But as we have shown in the chapters above, this work has been just like a drop in the ocean and there is so much more that urgently needs to be done.

In the light of our review, we formulate some recommendations concerning the methodology for conducting projects at a European level and present a set of guidelines for effective project management. These are in the boxes that follow (see Box 12.1 and Box 12.2). We are happy to disseminate here a declaration of the needs and rights of people with dementia and their carers. This declaration was first discussed at the Annual General Meeting of Alzheimer Europe in Lucerne, Switzerland (7-9 May, 1998). This declaration represents the voice of people with dementia in Europe and so we are reproducing it here in full. The declaration echoes many of the conclusions reached earlier in this book and we are pleased to be able to endorse it and disseminate it (see Box 12.3).

Final conclusion and recommendation

In the light of this review of the EC Alzheimer's projects we have seen that the European Commission has supported some significant new work in the field of dementia care. In terms of the wider scene of public health, however, this has been a minor activity with relatively small amounts of funding. In comparison to more "sexy" areas such as cancer and AIDS, the European Commission's Alzheimer's and dementia projects have been very small scale. The European Parliament has repeatedly called on the European Commission to adopt a full five-year programme of community action on Alzheimer's disease and other related disorders similar in scale to those adopted for cancer and AIDS. For whatever reason this has not happened.

The Amsterdam Treaty requires that the European Community should ensure that a high level of health protection is available to all European citizens. The European Commission has the political power to take any necessary actions to ensure that health protection is given to people with dementia and their carers. The time is right for the European Commission to give a maximum level of political recognition to the problem of dementia, to dementia sufferers and their carers.

The evidence reviewed in this book shows that there are many areas where dementia care can be improved. There is a need for:

- more support for informal carers
- more respite care facilities
- more expert centres
- more research on care settings, e.g. small housing units, group living
- more specialised care units
- more dementia services development units

- better professional training especially GPs, care workers, and volunteers
- standardisation of assessment and diagnostic procedures
- research on early assessment and diagnosis
- policies that promote equity of care
- closer co-ordination of health and social care

The European Commission should establish a Programme of Community Action on Alzheimer's disease and related disorders as a matter of priority. An Action Programme would be in accordance with the principle of health protection laid down in the Treaty of Amsterdam. The four million Europeans with dementia and their carers deserve no less. A European Programme of Community Action on dementia care would enable the above improvements to be carried out and other measures to be taken across the European Union. This would be a major and much needed step in dealing with dementia.

Box 12.1:   Recommendations on ADRD Project
                    Methodology

1   Obtain as large and as representative a sample of participants as possible.

2   If possible, randomly allocate participants to different treatment conditions or, at least, try to make sure that the participants in different conditions being compared are matched in order to reduce the influence of uncontrolled factors (minimising error). For example, if you are planning to compare groups (e.g. patients receiving different types of care, or carers living in

different countries) then make sure that they are matched for basic demographic and disease-related characteristics.

3   If possible, use both quantitative and qualitative methods of evaluation, as these tend to complement each other and relate to different aspects of the problem or issue, e.g. behavioural or medical outcomes vs. the experiences of caring.

4   Plan the design of your study or evaluation before you launch it.

5   Seek ethical guidance and apply for ethical clearance well before you begin to collect your data.

6   Consult a methodologist and/or statistician before you collect your data.

7   Pilot all questionnaires, interviews and methods before you begin your main study.

8   Use statistical methods that fit the kind of data you have collected.

9   Be careful not to over generalise your findings to groups, countries, cultures or populations outside of those studied.

10 In comparing your findings to those of others, methodological differences may be one of the reasons for any lack of agreement between different sets of findings.

Box 12.2: **Guidelines for Project Management of EC- funded ADRD Projects**

1 Avoid being overly ambitious; apply for an extension from Commission services if your project is getting behind its workplan.

2 Try to involve all partners equally; avoid artificial and opportunistic ("ghost") collaborators.

3 Meet with your collaborators at an early stage of the project to clarify the aims, terminology to be used, work timetable, and allocation of tasks and responsibilities.

4 Plan your work for the year and keep to deadlines.

5 Keep accurate records of your finances and time spent on the project.

6 Use sensitive terminology to describe people with ADRD, e.g. "people with dementia," not "demented people" or "the demented."

7 Disseminate your findings as widely as possible at conferences and workshops, in newspapers, magazines, books and journals.

8 Seek media attention for your project. If possible, obtain the assistance of the Press Office of your organisation and/or a professional Public Relations firm.

9 Be culturally sensitive.

10 Use professional translators. Supply the translators with a glossary of terms used in the field of ADRD.

11 Write a report that is clear, concise and user-friendly.

12 The size and weight of a report does not necessarily reflect its quality. In fact, the opposite is often the case. (We can state this with feeling!)

Box 12.3:   **Declaration of the needs and rights of people with dementia and their carers**

---

1   People with Alzheimer's disease or other dementia need:
- ◆   Accurate and timely diagnosis
- ◆   Information and understanding
- ◆   Health and social care

They have a right to be involved in decisions about their own lives, to protection under the law and to the best available health and social care in the country where they live.

2   Carers and family members need:
- ◆   Information and understanding
- ◆   Recognition of their special role and importance in the provision of care
- ◆   Identification of their own needs
- ◆   Provision of health and social care
- ◆   Financial support
- ◆   Carers and family members are essential to the care of people with dementia. They have a right to have their role recognised and to be consulted and involved in the provision of care and the development of services.

3   People with dementia need a range of health and social care provision:
- ◆   Accurate and timely diagnosis of treatable conditions
- ◆   Access to drug therapies on the basis of clinical use
- ◆   Access to neurological and psychiatric care from specialists

- Day care and home care services
- Respite for caregivers
- Sensitive and appropriate care for the dying

4   The social security and welfare systems of each country should ensure:
- Recognition of the financial costs of dementia to the person with dementia and their family
- Access to helpful benefits available in their country
- Financial support for younger people with dementia and their families
- Appropriate financial support for caregivers

5   Public awareness and education is the basis ofimproved care for people with dementia:
- Promotion of public understanding of dementia and the elimination of prejudice and discrimination
- Information for family caregivers
- Education for doctors and medical professionals
- Training for care workers and nurses

6   Research into the biological, clinical and psychological aspects of dementia is essential to improve care, develop therapies and ultimately find a treatment and cure:
- Research priorities should be directed towards the needs of people with dementia and their families
- Research should involve people with dementia and families as active participants
- Research should be ethical and acknowledge the importance of consent
- Research should aim for practical outcomes

7   Alzheimer Europe and its constituent members will achieve these aims by:

- Working in partnership with health and social care professionals
- Promoting the needs of people with dementia and their families to national governments and parliament
- Promoting the needs of people with dementia and their families to the European Parliament and Commission
- Sharing research, strategies, information and practice
- Encouraging and supporting caregivers and intergenerational solidarity
- Working together in respect for people with dementia and in ways that promote dignity, independence, choice and security

---

Source: Alzheimer Europe Newsletter, (1998)

GLOSSARY

Acetylcholine (ACh): a *neurotransmitter* that enables chemical messages to flow through the nervous system in memory and learning. Acetylcholine is severely reduced in Alzheimer's disease. Drugs to treat this deficit in the *cholinergic system* are used in treatment.

Acetylcholinesterase (AChE): an enzyme that breaks down acetylcholine after it has transmitted information between neurones. This enzyme is the main target for some anti-dementia drugs.

Acetylcholinesterase inhibitor (AChEI): a substance that prevents the normal degradation of acetylcholine by acetylcholinesterase. These substances are used as drugs to prolong the action of acetylcholine in the brain in AD patients.

Activities of Daily Living (ADL): ordinary everyday activities that may be affected by illness and that may be measured as an indicator of the level of handicap being experienced, e.g. walking up and down stairs, washing, dressing, toileting, etc.

AD: an abbreviation of "Alzheimer's disease."

ADRD: an abbreviation of "Alzheimer's disease and related disorders."

Allele: one or two or more different versions of the same gene.

Alzheimer Disease International (ADI): an international association of Alzheimer's disease carers involved in research, information exchange, advocacy, policy and services for people with ADRD with a head office in London.

Alzheimer Europe (AE): a federation of European Alzheimer's associations with a head office in Luxembourg.

Alzheimer's disease (AD): a progressive disease involving the destruction of nerve cells and the formation of *plaques* and *tangles* leading to severe dementia. It is the most common form of dementia.

Amyloid: a protein found in dense deposits forming the core of *plaques.* It builds up tissue in an amorphous way, and is one of the main features found in the brains of patients with AD.

Apolipoprotein (or Apoprotein): a protein bound to lipids in the bloodstream. Different forms of apolilipoprotein exist (ApoA, ApoB, ApoE, ...) each having a special role in transport and metabolism of lipids. ApoE4 is recognised as a risk factor of AD. This form of ApoE could influence the effect of drugs on AD.

Aricept (donepezil): a drug used to treat AD of the AChEI type.

Brain scan: a technique for examining the tissues and structures of the brain and central nervous system. A CT scan or MRI scan shows slices through the brain while a SPECT scan shows the brain's blood supply.

Care in the community: a term applied to the policy of some European Member States (e.g. Italy, UK) to provide care for people with disabilities and chronic illnesses outside of the hospital system.

Carer 'burden': a term used to describe the emotional and physical stresses and strains that accompany the care of people with chronic illnesses such as ADRD. An alternative term to describe this is *carer stress*.

Carer stress: the resulting effect or outcome of strain on carers of people suffering from illness. An alternative term for *carer 'burden'*.

Causal hypotheses: a scientific hypothesis that states that the cause of some process or condition X is another process or condition Y, e.g. that the AIDS syndrome is caused by the human immuno-deficiency virus (HIV). Controlled investigations that successfully eliminate other potential causes of the process or condition may test such hypotheses.

Cholinergic system: neurones emitting *acetylcholine* as a *neurotransmitter*.

Cognex (tacrine): a drug used to treat AD of the AChEI type.

Co-morbidity: the occurrence of two or more illnesses in the same person at the same time.

Continuum of care: the provision of a continuous standard or level of good care carried out with similar principles in the different settings in which the person being cared for lives, e.g. at home and in a day care centre.

Creutzfeldt-Jakob disease (CJD): a rare form of dementia caused by an infectious agent called a prion. It is introduced into the body by eating beef products contaminated by bovine spongiform encephalopathy (BSE) or "Mad Cow" Disease. Death occurs within about one year.

Cross-sectional survey: a survey that asks a group of people about their opinions or experiences at a particular point in time.

Dementia: a neurological disease that involves a decline of intellectual functions such as thinking, reasoning and remembering. Alzheimer's disease (AD) is the most common form of dementia.

Double-blind: a way of testing the efficacy of a drug treatment or intervention in which neither the investigator not the participants know which participants receive the drug and which receive a placebo (control).

DSM IV criteria: criteria developed in the USA for classifying patients with mental disorders into different diagnostic categories.

Equity: fairness or evenness in the access to, or availability and administration of services or resources across different population groups, e.g. men and women, Blacks and Whites, younger and older.

European Alzheimer's Clearing House (EACH): an organisation that aims to make better use of existing information and expertise (clearing) and to put forward "examples of good practice" in the field of care for patients with Alzheimer's Disease and Related Disorders (ADRD) with a head office in Brussels.

European Reminiscence Network: an organisation that promotes the use, study and value of reminiscence techniques in dementia and other forms of care with a head office in London.

Exelon® (rivastigmine): a drug used to treat AD of the AchEI type.

Expert centre: a centre of health professionals from many different disciplines (e.g. psychologists, gerontologists, psychiatrists, nurses, dieticians) who have the knowledge and skills necessary for the accurate diagnosis and effective care of people with dementia.

Folates: a nutrient found in foods as chicken liver, spinach, most breakfast cereals, orange and cauliflower.

Global deterioration scale (GDS): a widely used system for classifying the stages of intellectual decline in Alzheimer's disease developed by Barry Reisberg, an American neurologist.

Huntington's disease (Huntington's chorea): a hereditary disease occurring in middle age leading to dementia and involuntary twitching and muscle spasms.

Incidence: the number of new cases of an illness per year per 100,000 people in the population.

Informal care: care provided to a person suffering from disability, frailty and/or disease by family, friends and neighbours.

Korsakoff's syndrome: an alcohol related dementia that involves an irreversible loss of short-term memory.

Lewy-body disease: a type of dementia associated with abnormal collections of protein, known as Lewy-bodies, in the brain. People with this type of dementia show more daily variations in mental abilities than is typical of other forms of dementia.

Linoleic acid: a polyunsaturated fatty acid that may affect the development of cognitive impairment through its impact on atherosclerosis and thrombosis. A high intake of linoleic acid as low-density lipoprotein cholesterol may increase the risk of thrombosis and of dementia.

Memory aids: procedures for supporting the recall and conversation of people with dementia.

Mini Mental State Examination (or mini mental): a brief standardised method for assessing mental status using 11 items exploring memory, attention, calculation, language and praxis scored out of 30. In clinical trials patients with AD range from 12 to 23.

Multidisciplinary approach: acknowledges the need for management of ADRD using a team approach consisting of many professions, e.g. general practitioners, psychologists, specialists, nursing care, occupational therapy, social workers, support groups, Alzheimer's society, and respite/day care.

Multi-infarct dementia (MID): a form of dementia caused by many small strokes that gradually affect the functioning of the brain. This is the second most common form of dementia after AD.

Neurone: a nerve cell; the essential conducting unit of the nervous system consisting of a cell-body, dendrites, and one or more axons. A human brain consists of billions of neurones.

Neurotransmitter: a specialised chemical messenger that enables the flow of information through the nervous system. They are released by the axon of one neurone and excite or inhibit activity in neighbouring neurones. The concentration of several neurotransmitters is decreased in the brains of AD patients.

Parkinson's disease: a neurological disorder that is

characterised by slowness and loss of control of movements, a tremor and an expressionless face. It is associated with a loss of dopaminergic cells (cells using a *neurotransmitter* called dopamine) in the substantia nigra (a specific part of the brain).

Person centred approach: this is an approach to care of any type but to dementia care in particular that focuses upon the person, his or her individual personality, life history, likes and dislikes, needs, habits and interests. It was advocated by the late Tom Kitwood, an English psychologist. It is now widely considered to be the only really valid and humanistic approach to dementia care.

Pick's disease: a rare from of dementia that affects the frontal lobes of the brain.

Placebo: a substance that can be substituted for a drug but which has no specific activity used in drug trials.

Plaques: an unnatural occurrence of a matter called *amyloid* in the brain that forms plaques. Plaques interfere with the messages being sent from one nerve cell to another. They are found in the brains of people with AD.

Pre-senile dementia: an outmoded term for ADRD in a person who is under 65 years old.

Prevalence: the number of persons per 100,000 of the population with a particular illness at a particular time.

Prognosis: the prediction of the outcome of a disease.

Prospective design: a procedure that allows the causes of a condition to be studied by making observations over time, perhaps over several years, on a number of occasions on the same group of people. By taking a lot of different measurements the association between different outcomes or conditions that eventually occur with various earlier events and conditions can be studied. This design allows *causal hypotheses* to be tested.

Psychosocial interventions: treatments, therapies or counselling that are based on an understanding of the psychology and experience of people who have a particular illness.

Randomised: a method for allocating a drug or other treatment to patients based purely on chance (e.g. tossing a coin) used in controlled trials.

Reminiscence work: this involves the participants in acts of remembering or reminiscence that may be triggered by special objects of significance, songs, poems, pictures etc. It can have positive emotional effects through the restoration of group and personal identity among people with dementia.

Respite care: giving an informal carer a period of time off from their carer role.

Risk factor: an event or behaviour or condition that increases the probability that a particular disease will develop, e.g. eating a diet that is high in saturated fats and cholesterol is a risk factor for heart disease.

Senile dementia: an outmoded term for ADRD in a person who is 65 years or older.

Sense of coherence (SOC): a concept developed by the late Israeli medical sociologist, Aaron Antonovsky (1987). He defined SOC as a "global orientation that expresses the extent to which one has a pervasive, enduring though dynamic feeling of confidence that (1) the stimuli deriving from one's internal and external environments in the course of living are structured, predictable, and explicable; (2) the resources are available to one to meet the demands posed by these stimuli; and (3) these demands are challenges, worthy of investment and engagement."

Specialised care unit (SCU): a unit providing care to dementia patients that is dedicated to their particular needs and disabilities.

Synapse: the region where two or more neurones meet and impulses pass from one to the others.

Tangles: abnormal twisted cell fibres found in the bodies of neurones. These neurofibrillary tangles are found in the brains of AD patients.

Transmural care: providing professional care in community settings rather than in hospital.

USEFUL READING

Alzheimer Europe (1998)
Self-Help Carer Manual. Luxembourg. Published in Finnish, French German, Italian, Greek, Portuguese and English[09].

Cayton, H., Graham, N. & Warner, J. (1997)
Alzheimer's at Your Fingertips. London: Class Publishing.

Chapman, A. & Marshall, M. (Eds.), (1996)
Dementia: New Skills for Social Workers. London: Jessica Kingsley Publishers.

European Institute of Women's Health (1999)
Dementia Care. Challenges for an Ageing Europe. Dublin, Ireland.

Goldsmith, M. (1996)
Hearing the Voice of People with Dementia: Opportunities and Obstacles. London: Jessica Kingsley.

Kitwood, T. & Benson, S. (1995)
The New Culture of Dementia Care. London: Hawker Publications.

Kitwood, T. & Bredin, K. (1992)
Person to Person. Gale Centre Publications.

Mace, N.L., Rabins, P.V., Castleton, B.A., Cloke, C., & McEwan, E. (1985)
The Thirty Six Hour Day. London: Age Concern England.

Marshall, M. (1990)
Working with Dementia. Birmingham: Venture Press.

Useful Reading

Schweitzer, P. (1998)
Reminiscence in Dementia Care. London: Age Exchange[32].

SCIENTIFIC, MEDICAL AND TECHNICAL REPORTS

Antonovsky, A. (1987)
Unraveling the mystery of health. San Francisco: Jossey-Bass.

Baro, F., Haepers, K., Wagenfeld, M., & Gallagher, T. (1996)
Sense of coherence in caregivers to demented elderly persons in Belgium. In C. Stefanis & H. Hippius (Eds.) *Neuropsychology in old age: An update.* Seattle, WA: Hogrefe & Huber Publishers. Pp. 145-156.

Bianchetti, A., Benvenutii, P, Ghisla, K.M., Frisoni, G.B., & Trabucchi, M. (1997)
An Italian model of dementia special care unit: Results of a pilot study. *Alzheimer's Disease and Associated Disorders*, 11, 53-56.

Boothby, H. et al. (1997)
National policy needs to be set for prescribing of this drug (donepezil). *British Medical Journal*, 315, 1623.

Bourgeois, M.S. (1990)
Enhancing conversation skills in patients with Alzheimer's disease using a prosthetic memory aid. *Journal of Applied Behavioral Analysis*, 23, 31-64.

Bourgeois, M.S. (1992)
Evaluating memory wallets in conversations with persons with dementia. *Journal of Speech and Hearing Research*, 35, 1344-1357.

Bourgeois, M.S. (1993)
Effects of memory aids on the dyadic conversations of

individuals with dementia. *Journal of Applied Behavior Analysis*, 26, 77-87.

Brodaty, H., Howarth, G.C., Mant, A., & Kurrle, S.E. (1994)
General practice and dementia: A national survey of Australian GPs. *Medical Journal of Australia*, 160, 10-14.

Bryant, C.A., Ouldred, E. & Jackson, S.H.D. (1998)
Purpuric rash with donepezil treatment. *British Medical Journal*, 317, 787.

Communication from the Commission of the European Communities on Development of Public Health Policy in the European Community, Brussels, 15 April, 1998.

Corey-Bloom, J., Anand, R. & Veach, J. for the ENA 713 B352 Study Group (1998).
A randomised trial evaluating the efficacy and safety of ENA 713 (rivastigmine tartrate), a new acetylcholinesterase inhibitor, in patients with mild to moderately severe Alzheimer's disease. *International Journal of Geriatric Psychopharmacology*, 1, 55-65.

Frisoni, G.B., Gozzetti, A., Bignamini, V., Vellas, B.J., Berger, A.K., Bianchetti, A., Rozzinin, R., & Trabucchi, M. (1998)
Special care units for dementia in nursing homes: A controlled study of effectiveness. *Archives of Gerontology and Geriatrics*, 6, 215-224.

Grahn, G. (1998)
Leva med demens-handikapp. Drottningholm, Sweden: Stiftelsen Silvihemmet.

Hamilton, M. (1960)
A rating scale for depression. *Journal of Neurology, Neurosurgery and Psychiatry*, 12, 56-62.

Heinrich, R. (1998)
All or nothing in case of Alzheimer's? European recommendations for diagnosis and therapy of dementia. Bayer Satellite Symposium, 8th European Meeting, Alzheimer Europe, Lucerne, Switzerland, May, 1998.

Heller, T. & Factor, A. (1991)
Permanency planning for adults with mental retardation living with family caregivers. *American Journal on Mental Retardation*, 96, 163-176.

Hindmarch, I., Lehfeld, H., de Jongh, P., & Erzigkeit, H. (1998)
The Bayer Activities of Daily Living Scale (B-ADL). *Dementia and Geriatric Cognitive Disorders*, 9(supplement), 20-24.

Holden, R.J. (1999)
Could a high cholesterol diet cause Alzheimer's disease in Western society? *Human Psychopharmacology*, 14, 185-188.

Hurley, A.C., Volicer, B., Mahoney, M.A., Volier, L. (1993)
Palliative fever management in Alzheimer patients. Quality plus fiscal responsibility. Advances in *Nursing Science*, 16: 21-23

Jerrom, B., Mian, I. & Rukanyake, N.G. (1993)
Stress on the relative caregivers of dementia sufferers, and predictors of the breakdown of community care. *International Journal of Geriatric Psychiatry*, 8, 331-337.

Jones, R.W., Mann, J. & Saunders, S.A. (1997)
Prices charges for private prescriptions for donepezil show huge variation. *British Medical Journal*, 315, 1623.

Kalmijn, S. (1997)
Risk factors for cognitive decline. Doctoral dissertation, Erasmus University, Rotterdam.

Launer, L.J. et al (1999)
Rates and risk factors for dementia and Alzheimer's disease. Results from EURODEM pooled analyses. *Neurology*, 52, 78-84.

Linn, M.W. & Linn, B.S. (1982)
The Rapid Disability Rating Scale-2. *Journal of the American Geriatrics Society*, 30, No. 8.

Marks, D.F. (1998)
The major complaints of carers. Bayer Satellite Symposium, 8th European Meeting, Alzheimer Europe, Lucerne, Switzerland, May, 1998.

Marks, D.F., Murray, M., Evans, B. & Willig, C. (2000)
Health Psychology: Theory, Research & Application. London: Sage (in press).

Marks, D.F., Pitt, C., Thomas, S., & Sykes, C.M. (1999)
Caring for a family member with dementia: a psychological study of stress, strain and sense of coherence. In preparation.

Novartis (1998)
Product Monograph. Exelon (rivastigmine). Cheshire, England: Gardiner-Caldwell Communications Ltd.

Ott, A. (1997)
Risk of dementia. Doctoral dissertation, Erasmus University, Rotterdam.

Pearlin, L.I., Mullan, J.T., Semple, S.J., & Skaff, M.M. (1990)
Caregiving and the stress process: An overview of concepts and their measures. *Gerontologist,* 30, 583-594.

Reisberg, B. et al. (1982)
The global deterioration scale for assessment of primary degenerative dementia. *American Journal of Psychiatry,* 139, 1136-1139.

Rogers, S.L., Farlow, M.R., Mohr, R., Friedhoff, L.T. and the Donepezil Study Group (1998)
A 24 week double blind, placebo-controlled trial of donepezil in patients with Alzheimer's disease. *Neurology, 50,* 136-145.

Roth, M. et al. (1986)
CAMDEX, a standardised instrument for the diagnosis of mental disorder in the elderly with special reference to early detection of dementia. *British Journal of Psychiatry,* 149, 698-709.

Slooter, A.J.C. (1998)
The role of apolipoprotein E in atherosclerosis and dementia. Doctoral dissertation, Erasmus University, Rotterdam.

Stein, K., Milne, R. & Best, L. (1997)
More convincing evidence of efficacy needs to be cited. *British Medical Journal,* 315, 1623.

Stewart, A., Phillips, R. & Dempsey, G. (1998)
Pharmacotherapy for people with Alzheimer's Disease: A

Markov model of five years therapy using donepezil. *International Journal of Geriatric Psychiatry*, 13, 445-453.

Volicer, L., Collard, A. Hurley, A., Bishop, C. Kern, D., Karon, S. (1994)
Impact of special care for patients with advanced Alzheimer's disease on patients' discomfort and cost. *Journal of American Geriatric Society*, 42, 597-603.

Walker, A. (1995)
Integrating the family into mixed economy of care. *The future of family care for older people*, (Eds.) Allen, I and Perkins, E. London: HMSO.

Wimo, A., Adolfsson, R., Sandman, P.O. (1994)
The impact of cognitive decline and workload on the costs of dementia care. *International Journal of Geriatric Psychiatry*, 9, 479-484.

Wimo, A., Wallin, J. Lundgren, K. et al (1991)
Group living, an alternative for dementia patients – a cost analysis. *International Journal of Geriatric Psychiatry*, 6, 21-29.

Zarit, S.H., Orr, N.K., Zarit, J.M. (1985)
The hidden victims of Alzheimer's Disease. New York: New York University Press.

USEFUL ADDRESSES

Alzheimer Associations in the European Union

Country	Organisation/Executive Director
Austria	Alzheimer Angehörige Austria Obere Augartenstraße 26-28 1020 Vienna, Austria Tel: +43 1 332 5166 Fax: +43 1 334 2141 E-mail: alzheimeraustria@via.at
Belgium	National Alzheimer Liga Mr Van Daele, 39 Watertorenlaan 1831 Machelen, Belgium
Belgium (Dutch- Sector)	Alzheimer Liga Stationstraat 60-62 2300 Turnhout, Belgium Tel: +32 14 43 5060 Fax: +32 14 43 7654
Belgium (French/ German- Sectors)	Ligue Alzheimer Clinique Le Perî 4B rue Montagne Ste Walburge 4000 Liege, Belgium Tel: +32 4 225 8793 Fax: +32 4 226 7231
Denmark	Alzheimerforeningen Skt Lukas Vej 13, DK - 2900 Hellerup Denmark

	Tel: +45 39 40 0488
	Fax: +45 39 61 6699

Finland	Alzheimer-Keskusliitto
	Ms Varpu Kettunen
	Luotsikatu 4 E, 00160 Helsinki, Finland
	Tel: +358 9 622 6200
	Fax: +358 9 62 26 2020
	E-mail: varpu.kettunen@alzheimer.fi

France	Association France Alzheimer
	Mr Arnaud Fraiss
	21, Boulevard Montmartre, 75002 Paris
	France
	Tel: +33 1 42 97 5241
	Fax: +33 1 42 96 0470

Germany	Deutsche Alzheimer Gesellschaft
	Ms Sabine Jansen,
	Kantstr. 152, 10623 Berlin, Germany
	Tel: +49 30 3150 5733
	Fax: +49 30 3150 5735
	E-mail: deutsche.alzheimer.ges@
	t-online.de

Greece	Greek Alzheimer Association
	Ms Magda Tsolaki
	Macri 16, Sikies Thessaloniki
	G-56625, Greece
	Tel: +30 31 350 332
	Fax: +30 31 357 603

Ireland	Alzheimer Society of Ireland
	Mr Norman Stuart

Alzheimer House
43, Nothumberland Avenue
Dún Laoghaire, Co. Dublin, Ireland
Tel: +353 1 284 6616
Fax: +353 1 284 6030
E-mail: alzheimer@iol.ie

Italy	A.I.M.A. Ripa di Porta Ticinese 21, 20143 Milano Italy Tel: +39 02 8940 6254 Fax: +39 02 8940 4192 E-mail: aimanaz@tin.it
Italy	Federazione Alzheimer Italia Via Marino 7, 20121 Milan, Italy Tel: +39 02 80 9767 Fax: +39 02 87 5781 E-mail: alzit@mbox.vol.it Website: www.alzheimer.it
Luxembourg	Ms Camilla Goetschalckx Association Luxembourg Alzheimer B.P. 5021, L-1050 Luxembourg Luxembourg Tel: +352 42 1676 Fax: +352 42 1679 E-mail: ala@selection-line.net Website: www.alzheimer-europe.org/luxembourg
Netherlands	Alzheimerstichting Harry A. Crielaars

Postbus 183, 3980 CD Bunnik
The Netherlands
Tel: +31 30 659 6285
Fax: +31 30 659 6283
E-mail: info@alzheimer-ned.nl
Website: www.alzheimer-ned.nl

Portugal	APFADA Apartado 14319, 1064 Lisboa, Portugal Tel: +351 1 353 34 94 Fax: +351 1 353 3494
Spain	Fundación Alzheimer España Rafael Salgado, 7-1° dcha 28036 Madrid, Spain Tel: +34 91 457 8725 Fax: +34 91 457 9542 E-mail: ALZHEURO@LANDER.ES Website: www.eurociber.es/solitel/alzheimer
Sweden	Alzheimerföreningen i Sverige Sunnanväg 14 S, 222 26 Lund, Sweden Tel: +46 46 14 7318 Fax: +46 46 18 8976 E-mail: Alzheimf@algonet.se Website: www.psykiatr.lu.se/alzheim/
Sweden	Demensförbundet Mr Sten-Sture Lidén Drakenbergsgatan 13 nb 117 41 Stockholm, Sweden Tel: +46 8 658 5222

Fax: +46 8 658 6068
E-mail: rdr@demensforbundet.se
Website: www.demensforbundet.se

United Kingdom	Alzheimer's Disease Society
	Harry Cayton, Exec. Director
	Gordon House, 10 Greencoat Place
	London SW1 1PH
	Tel: +44 171 306 0606
	Fax: +44 171 306 0808
	E-mail: info@alzheimers.org.uk
	Website: www.alzheimers.org.uk
United Kingdom	Mr. Jim Jackson
	Alzheimer Scotland-Action on Dementia
	22 Drumsheugh Gardens
	Edinburgh EH3 7RN
	Tel: +44 131 243 1453
	Fax: +44 131 243 1450
	E-mail: alzheimer@alzscot.org
	Website: www.alzscot.org

General Useful Addresses

Alzheimer's Disease International
45/46 Lower Marsh
London, SE1 7RL, UK
Tel: +44 171 620 3011
Fax: +44 171 401 7351

Dementia Services Development Centre
University of Stirling
Stirling, FK9 4LA
Tel: +44 1786 467 740
Fax: +44 1786 466846

European Commission Services
EC DG V/F/3 Bâtiment Jean Monnet
Plateau du Kirchberg, L-2920
Luxembourg
Tel: +352 4301 1
Fax: +352 4301 34511

Middlesex University Health Research Centre
Queensway, Enfield, Middlesex
EN3 4SF, UK
Tel/Fax: +44 181 362 5558
